THE ORIGINAL
NATURAL HYGIENE
WEIGHT-LOSS DIET BOOK

The Original

::::::::::::::::::::::::::::::::::::::

NATURAL HYGIENE
WEIGHT-LOSS
DIET BOOK

::

by

HERBERT M. SHELTON, D.P., N.D.,

JO WILLARD and JEAN A. OSWALD

Keats Publishing, Inc. ▓ New Canaan, Connecticut

The Original Natural Hygiene Weight-Loss Diet Book
Copyright © 1986 by Jo Willard, Jean A. Oswald
and Willowdeen Rosner
ISBN: 0-87983-376-9
Library of Congress Catalog Card Number: 86–2767
Printed in the United States of America

KEATS PUBLISHING, INC.
27 Pine Street, New Canaan, Connecticut 06840

NOTE: This book is not intended as a substitute for receiving professional medical or Hygienic advice. The weight-loss program is not designed for women who are pregnant or who are breast-feeding. The three-day fast is not recommended to those with diabetes or tuberculosis or to those who are taking drugs. Check with your doctor before starting this or any other diet plan.

To Herbert M. Shelton
who revived and refined
the philosophy and science
of Natural Hygiene
and who died on January 1, 1935
too soon to see this book in print.

CONTENTS

....

THE AUTHORS

DR. HERBERT M. SHELTON

October 6, 1895–January 1, 1985

HERBERT M. SHELTON was born in Wylie, Texas. In 1920, he received a doctorate in physiological therapeutics from the International College of Drugless Physicians in Chicago. In 1924, he completed a doctorate from the American School of Chiropractic and a doctorate from the American School of Naturopathy, New York City. While in New York he taught courses in dietetics and naturopathic principles at the American School of Naturopathy.

Dr. Shelton worked as a staff writer for Bernarr MacFadden's *Physical Culture* magazine, as a health columnist for the *New York Evening Graphic*, and as editor of *How to Live,* and published his own monthly magazine called *Dr. Shelton's Hygienic Review* for forty-one years. Dr. Shelton was one of the primary influences in organizing the American Natural Hygiene Society and in 1949 was elected its first president. He taught the Hygienic program of living to over 30,000 health seekers who sought his care at all three of his health schools in San Antonio, Texas, between 1928 and 1981.

Dr. Shelton, a preeminent authority on dietetics and

author of over forty books, died peacefully in his sleep at his home in Alamo Heights, Texas, in January 1985.

JO WILLARD

JO WILLARD's career was interrupted in her late twenties and early thirties when she was diagnosed as having arthritis and stomach ulcers, along with a myriad of other symptoms.

Years of medical supervision and drugs only aggravated the symptoms until she was urged to "learn to live with it." Robbed of hope and help, Jo turned to "alternative health modalities."

Each new concept gave her more hope for healing and a new perception of disease, but not until she discovered Natural Hygiene did she find the philosophical and scientific thread of her life: *taking responsibility for what happens to you.*

With new hope and increasing knowledge, her health improved and at age forty-eight she returned to school, studying engineering and later the humanities.

Her vocation as manager and secretary-treasurer of a company manufacturing mechanical components became a counterpoint to her avocation of teaching the principles of natural health care.

Since becoming aware of how the body and mind function and learning what is required to keep well, Jo has dedicated her life to promoting and teaching the techniques for freedom from illness, freedom from the fear of illness, and avoidance of the exploitation of the sick. She is particularly interested in exposing any political corruption of various agencies entrusted with people's health.

Jo was elected first vice-president of the American Hygiene Society and served as the Society's first executive director for three years as well as being active on its executive board for many years. She has also served as president of the Connecticut Chapter of the American Natural Hygiene Society since 1970.

Today, Jo is the president of Natural Hygiene, Inc., a non-profit educational organization, and is a member of the advisory board of the University of Bridgeport Institute for Nutrition. She has produced a weekly radio talk show on Natural Hygiene since 1973, and now also produces a Natural Hygiene television program.

She has lectured extensively throughout the United States and Canada and is considered one of the most foremost twentieth-century Hygienic teachers.

JEAN A. OSWALD

JEAN A. OSWALD was born in Hales Corners, Wisconsin. She attended Carthage College, Kenosha, Wisconsin, on a scholarship and graduated from the University of Wisconsin with a degree in education in 1971. Afterward, she worked as an artist, teacher and freelance writer.

In 1977, Jean suffered from an asthmatic condition caused by smoking cigarettes and exposure to asbestos, nitric acid, sulphuric acid and molten toxic fumes while working with jewelry and ceramics. She fasted twenty-eight days at Dr. Scott's Natural Hygiene Institute, Cleveland, Ohio, and thereafter adopted a Hygienic lifestyle. Her recovery and experiences resulted in a book coauthored with Dr. Shelton titled *Fasting For The Health of It*. The book, published in 1983, included one hundred case histories of fasts documented from the cumulative experiences of eleven Hygienic practitioners who had supervised a total of 200,000 fasts over a period of sixty years.

Presently, Jean is teaching in the Milwaukee public school system and finishing work on a biography of Dr. Shelton. She lives with her husband, Jim, in Franklin, Wisconsin.

ACKNOWLEDGMENTS

Our most sincere gratitude is expressed to Dr. Gerald Benesh, not only for writing the Foreword but for offering his authoritative comments and suggestions; to Willowdeen Rosner, Jim Oswald and Walden Shelton for their continual support and assistance; to Loretta Steckhan for her expert typing and advice; to Dr. Sharon Dedinas and Constance Corcoran for their valuable editorial assistance; and to Dr. Monroe Burton, Dr. Ralph Cinque and Dr. Frank Sabatino, who gave their critical appraisal of the views presented in this book.

Many, many warm thanks to Dr. Bernard and Kate Sharp; Ida Shelton; Roger, Dores and Rhonda Steckhan; Erma Benesh; and Anita Reuter for their useful assistance in the preparation of this book.

Foreword

WRITING the foreword to this book is indeed a great pleasure and honor.

The information in the book is long overdue, not because there is a shortage of books on the subject—on the contrary, there is a plethora of books and articles, nearly all of them misleading. Radio and television shows add to the confusion.

Counting calories, lopsided diets and feasting followed by fasting only further upsets the already inharmonious state of the individual. The raised consciousness of vegetarians and naturalists has floundered in this sea of misinformation. But there is a definitive, scientific approach to the concepts of health and weight loss, concepts which are too often misunderstood.

A simpler, more natural approach is the need of the hour. This book on losing weight meets this historic need. The authors approach this serious problem from a rational, knowledgeable point of view, taking into account all the basic involvements of biochemistry, psychology and Nature. They are dedicated people who approach the project from the basics of the natural laws of life—meeting the biochemical needs of the body and mind.

Society has imbued us with perverted habits not conducive to health. The authors of this book clearly present a better way of life, not simply a diet to assuage or remedy the symptoms of obesity. Their book reveals secrets of living in accord with God's natural laws. This informative volume is filled with basic facts on the subject of living the good life.

Eating should and must be pleasurable, but not at the expense of injury to vital structures which leads to sickness and death. Eating is one of life's greatest pleasures. It can become even more pleasurable as one regains health.

In every century, a personality arises who is destined to change the course of life for many people. In the twentieth century, this man was Dr. Herbert M. Shelton, whose life was dedicated to truth. A fearless man of great stature, he often said and wrote "Let us have Truth though the heavens fall." He spent many hours laboring for humankind, collecting old volumes of material which were written by authors who also searched far and wide to bring facts of living a healthful life to the people.

Dr. Shelton often quoted and gave credit to these former great ones who laid a foundation upon which Natural Hygiene as we know it today was built. He took no credit for his efforts, but always honored the work of his predecessors.

As a young man I was deeply impressed by Dr. Shelton's sincerity and desire to promote Natural Hygiene. He had no tolerance for frauds or promoters whose chief motivations were prestige and monetary gains. Dr. Shelton was truly dedicated to the promotion of health truth and fully realized the great potential that the Creator instilled in all of us. He rarely mentioned God in his writings, but fully realized the innate power that we possess and acknowledged this infinite power which resides in every cell of our beings. He gave credit and credence to this vital force.

Dr. Shelton always spoke of the laws of life which govern and control all life in all living things. This primal consideration was the triggering mechanism which caused me to realize that only Nature (the body) heals itself and has the inherent power to do so. And it was the realization of this fact that caused me to accept the principles of Natural Hygiene completely.

It has been my experience with obese or overweight persons that they may have a deeply hidden dislike of themselves (as they are). Eating, or I should say overeating, is an escape mechanism they employ that camouflages this feeling. It can be termed a substitution. Obese people do not like what they see in the mirror. What they view creates a greater lack of self-esteem, and they love themselves less as time goes on. Therefore, their minds must first of all be changed before other measures are taken. This is a time when a complete fast plays a primary role in the program.

The fast provides the opportunity for self-evaluation, a time for introspection. It is the best opportunity for a complete inventory of past life and future direction, and perhaps the first time for a clear view of self.

As the cells of the body change from bad to better, the psyche also changes. Each cell is a conscious organism directly and indirectly controlled by the mind. Thoughts do influence cell and body function and the reverse is also true.

You can readily see how important the proper use of your mind is in life's processes, whether you are thin, overweight or of normal weight. How you think and what you think of yourself are prime considerations. Without accepting this, you are sure to fail.

Rewards in overcoming obesity are many. They include greater self-respect, greater love of self, greater ability to love others, greater reverence for life itself, and above all, a greater realization of what and who you really are. To experience the exuberance, energy and joy of health, rise to the challenge, for within each of us resides a greatness that needs only to be released. Truly, a sleeping giant is waiting to serve you.

Wake up to this change and claim your rightful place on this earth.

GERALD BENESH, D.C., N.D.

Introduction

THIS BOOK is written at a time when a profusion of "winning diets" and often *harmful* weight-loss diets confound and confuse the public. Even though awareness of health issues is growing in our society, people today are disease-ridden, primarily with degenerative diseases.

It is a time of change—qualitative change and quantitative change. It is a time of raised consciousness, of searching for alternatives. Perhaps at no time in history have people had a more profound assignment, a more profound responsibility to themselves, to their families and to every human being.

By assisting at age eighty-eight in the writing of this book, Dr. Herbert M. Shelton rendered a great service to humanity and fulfilled a great need. This timely book on losing weight and eating for high-level health meets that need, for it provides a total program of superior nutrition that supplies all the requisites for healthy physiology.

Dr. Shelton rediscovered and revived the science and philosophy called Natural Hygiene. The Natural Hygiene system of health care teaches the conditions of health and points out how disease is built. It was through Dr. Shelton's dedicated efforts, his teachings, his writings, his publications and his leadership that Natural Hygiene was again brought to the attention of people who have been drugged, physically and psychologically—drugged to believe that what is allowed to be sold as food is adequate wherewithal for the "replacement parts" of the body.

A book on diet usually draws from widely different sources. Dr. Shelton has drawn from Nature's laws—from knowledge of the basic biochemical needs of the body, and from his sixty-five years of devotion and dedication to people's health. Dr. Shelton used his researched knowledge of Nature to guide scores of thousands of people carefully, intelligently and lovingly back to health in his famous Hygienic Institute, Dr. Shelton's Health School in San Antonio, Texas. It was here that he tested, refined and observed the application of all the laws to fit the individual needs of the sick and obese.

Dr. Shelton's work encompasses a conspectus of Nature's laws, from the vegetarianism of Pythagoras and Einstein to the reminder that food is one and only one aspect of the circumstances which create health. The role of food in good health must be viewed in relation to all other aspects of the laws of Nature.

Dr. Shelton's work makes a special contribution in its definitive exposure of the politics of food. He defies the social structure by exposing its callous attitudes towards people's health.

The science and philosophy of Natural Hygiene work. The "Wellness" movement, the "Wholistic Health" movement, all work only to the degree that they embrace Natural Hygiene. Natural Hygiene is not a fad, a movement or an organization, but an awakening consciousness that our society and its mores are not geared to our health. To the degree that your consciousness is raised, to the degree that you break with the social poisons, to the degree that you become autonomous in your lifestyle, to the degree that you program your own inherent computer, to that degree will you be free from the symptoms of dis-ease.

In changing your lifestyle and eating for high-level health, wonderful fringe benefits are achieved—beauty of the face and body. Your body finds its correct weight for your frame and redistributes the weight intelligently, based on its inner wisdom and your genetic proclivities. *Result: an ideal weight,* clear and beautiful complexion, and a *joie de vivre* that endows you with a sense of wellbeing and high energy.

The dieting program presented in this book is not new. The origins of this diet, in conjunction with the philosophy of Natural Hygiene, date back to the 1830s when a courageous Hygienist, Sylvester Graham, advocated a vegetarian diet despite great opposition to his revolutionary reform. In 1890, Hygienist Emmet Densmore, M.D. became a follower of Graham and added his knowledge of food combining to the vegetarian program. In 1912, physiologist Ivan Pavlov made significant contributions. Eight years later, Hygienist John H. Tilden, M.D., although he was not a vegetarian, contributed the idea of eating proteins and starches at separate meals. Today, more than sixty years of experience have gone into improving and perfecting this dietary program.

Portions of the information in this book have been condensed from Dr. Shelton's *Food and Feeding* (1926), *The Natural Diet of Man* (1931), *The Hygienic System— Orthotropy* (1935), *Health for the Millions* (1968), and *Food Combining Made Easy* (revised edition 1982). The latest book, *Food Combining Made Easy*, has been translated into Greek, Italian, Spanish, Swedish, French, Hindi and Portuguese. An estimated half-million people have found success through following the Hygienic way of eating and living.

This book can prompt you to take a giant leap forward in your life, not only physically but emotionally. Indeed, it is a giant step forward in your total evolvement.

We remain forever grateful and honored to have worked on this book with Dr. Shelton, one of the greatest health educators of all time.

JO WILLARD
JEAN A. OSWALD

PART ONE

....

SET THE COURSE FOR SUCCESS

The only successful weight-loss program is one that is in tune with an individual's nutritional needs and his/her physical and mental wellbeing.

ROBERT S. MENDELSOHN, M.D.
Author and health advocate

CHAPTER ONE

GETTING YOUR MIND AND BODY IN THE RIGHT PERSPECTIVE

A SPECIFIC ITEM cannot be singled out to blame for causing over 50 percent of the population to be overweight. The total diet, as eaten today, is faulty. Not only does it contain excess proteins, fats, sugar, and starch, but it is made up largely of refined and processed foods, foods that have been artificially flavored, colored, preserved and adulterated. In addition, these foods are too often eaten in haphazard, indigestible combinations. This book calls for an all-out approach to the present-day need for total reform of weight-loss dieting, with an emphasis on correct food combining.

Here are testimonials from a few of the thousands of people who have tested this approach.

"I look younger . . . and feel younger."
"My complexion has taken on a new glow. . . ."

"My blood pressure, cholesterol and triglyceride
levels are lower. . . ."
"I have more energy . . . I feel like a human
dynamo. . . ."

"Breathing is easier . . . I move with greater ease."
"My mind is clearer and sharper."
"No more acid indigestion . . . no more gas . . . no
constipation. . . ."
"My insomnia is gone."
"I have a new lease on life . . . and I'm interested
in sex again."
"My senses are keener . . . my taste buds re-
fined. . . ."
"I have more efficient digestion and assimilation. . . ."
"My overall wellbeing is vastly improved. I feel
reborn."
"I lost twenty pounds in one month and most
important, *I kept it off.*"

Weight-loss testimonies vary. We cannot guarantee
how much you will lose. This depends on your sex
(men tend to lose weight a bit faster than women),
how overweight you are to begin with, and your activity schedule. Naturally, it's hard to compare two different people who are slimming. If one is active, the other
sedentary, the latter's rate will, of course, be slower.
But it is safe to say you can expect to lose from twelve
to twenty-four pounds by following the plan for one
month. And remember that your success is not measured only by the absolute amount of pounds you lose.
Your overall physical wellbeing will improve from eating better foods, and your emotional wellbeing will

improve when you recognize the source of your overeating.

If this sounds good to you, let's get started. Keep in mind your desire to feel good and be healthy. Believe you deserve it and that you can discover the beautiful person you are!

In general, three things happen when you eat more food than your body immediately needs:

1. Much of the food passes in an undigested state into the colon and is eliminated by normal bowel action. Sometimes laxatives, enemas or colonics are resorted to, which ultimately cause more problems.

2. Some of the food is expelled in the urine, or through the mucous membranes as mucus.

3. Some food may be stored as fat.

Now, what harm does this do to your mind and body? The habit of taking excess food and taking wrong foods in wrong combinations clouds your mind and depresses your body's precious energies. Work is a burden, *living* is a burden, and tasks take twice as long as they should. Since wrong eating habits waste your energy and retard or destroy your development, they must be considered as self-destructive.

In the following excerpt, Hygienist Stanley S. Bass, D.C., explains exactly how the body reacts when huge masses of food are eaten. Many people use excess eating as a stimulant:

> The exciting lust for food varieties, tastes, and excessive eating (even of the best foods), whips the body into action of intensified digestion, absorption and assimilation. While it is stimulating and exciting at first, as we overload with food, it acts as a

narcotic depressant secondarily and stupefies the mind and emotions. Hence its popularity and frequent use as an escape mechanism from emotional problems by compulsive overeaters who turn their feeling, emotions and thoughts off by literally stupefying their brain cells. The immense labor needed to digest this huge mass of food draws most of the blood away from the brain to the stomach. The brain experiences a secondary type of anemia, causing the inducement of a very drowsy state, and frequently long hours of sleep are needed to recuperate from this awesome digestive burden.

If vital energies are dissipated instead of being conserved, you will age faster and exhaust both your mind and your body. When less work is imposed upon the digestive organs, energy is conserved and available for other purposes. Thus, following our plan of wholesome eating will result in healthful energy conservation. You are guaranteed better health than you had when you started the program.

DEVELOP A LUST FOR LIVING

People rarely want to be fat. With increased weight, various forms of disease evolve more easily. Yet only 15 percent of all dieters who lose weight are able to retain their weight loss, regardless of the program followed. What happens to the 85 percent who backslide into a slow form of suicide? The answer lies in a spiritual maladjustment, habits of negative thinking and inadequate health awareness.

People often grow fat and diseased because of an inability to cope with situations that confront them. The villain is circumstance—there is often the pressure to eat. You become conditioned to using food as a catalyst for many occasions, or as a substitute for love, or because you are bored or angry. You can replace feelings of boredom, anger, worry, disappointment, guilt, fear, self-pity, resentment and hostility, with feelings of joy, contentment, peace of mind and love, coupled with productive activity. Learning to use your natural, inherent powers for life instead of powers for death will set you free from overeating. Refusing to allow destructive habits and thoughts to rule you will bring you unerringly to your goal of permanent weight loss. The result is improved health and a longer, more abundant life.

Losing weight requires a healthy attitude toward your inner self, your spiritual nature. Your mind's eye *must* capture the image of a new slender body. A poor self-image is more fattening than rich carbohydrates because you will repeatedly eat "junk food" as long as you are not more tender and loving to yourself. All excesses, whether of eating, drinking or smoking, have roots in your attitudes, your thoughts and your emotions. You cannot get rid of the excesses without first getting rid of the cause. If you conceive of yourself as spiritually well adjusted, perfectly in tune with the legitimate needs of your body, you will soon achieve physical improvement. You must understand that the success of this weight-loss program will become manifest when you break away from self-destructive habits. Turn them into constructive health habits of feeling and living. It is not so much what is in your refrigerator, although that is very important, but what is in your mind. Your physical health proceeds from mental peace, while self-destructive habits proceed from mental confusion, discontentment and unhappiness.

Take a spiritual approach to losing weight naturally. Recognize the seven emotional needs that prompt overeating. Find yours and work on it!

1. Need for love
2. Need for a good time
3. Need for happiness
4. Need to escape from reality
5. Need to feel free from anxiety
6. Need to overcome life depression
7. Need to get rid of anger

If you approach this diet with the thought of merely cutting down on your food intake, this will not necessarily make you thinner *permanently*. Like taking a tranquilizer if you lose your job, it is a temporary measure and in no way tackles the underlying problem. You must learn who you are, how you function and why you do certain things. You lose weight with your head more than with or without food. The desire for food is simply a need for emotional and spiritual gratification. Get the real thing and your need for extra food vanishes.

To reach your goal of permanent weight loss, cultivate happiness and laughter with as much care and persistency as the gardener gives to his plants. Happiness and laughter promote digestion, color the cheeks, put a sparkle in your eyes and buoyancy in your tread. Dr. Wayne Dyer, in *Your Erroneous Zones,* asserts that the absence of laughter indicates pathology. He says, "Perhaps the single most outstanding characteristic of healthy people is their unhostile sense of humor. Helping others choose to laugh, and learning to stand back and observe the incongruity of almost every life situation is an excellent remedy for anger." Happiness and laughter are traits you have the ability to choose when you want to.

Without happiness, your emotional misery affects other physical aspects of your life as well. Food often disagrees with unhappy people, and their bowels seldom function properly. They seldom sleep well and they may continually discover new symptoms, new pains and new worries. Unfortunately, the repeated taking of excess food to cope with problems of living provides only a temporary "pleasure," followed by greater unhappiness. Loss of weight cannot be achieved in unhappiness. You must choose happiness, dismiss your troubles and think about the better things in life. Having people to love, something to do and something to look forward to will increase your happiness. And this happiness will result in improved digestion and improved assimilation.

But a joyous state of mind is not the only prerequisite for beginning a weight-loss program. Happiness is not without cause. It is a product: it is the result of a life well lived. To elevate happiness as the foundation of health is inadequate and lopsided. For an obese person, it would be foolish to say if you will simply become happy you will get thin. Happiness must be combined with knowledge of good nutrition. In the very nature of things, there can be no such thing as good health with very bad nutrition. Nor can there be good nutrition in a profoundly unhappy person. In a very wide sense, happiness and health are almost synonymous terms, and the two states are dependent upon each other.

Your inner, intuitive voice is your guide. It should never be confused with the ego, or "strident voice." When in doubt, quiet your body and mind—let go of any investment in your answer and listen to that still, small, peaceful and loving voice within. It is the authentic voice. When you learn to make this distinction, you will be filled with an incredible sense of security and inner strength.

You have the power within you to choose to be happy and slim or unhappy and fat. You must recognize that the same power within you can bring either health and happiness or sorrow and sickness. This power exists in *every man and woman*. Every condition and circumstance in your life can be changed by this inherent power. Draw upon it and learn to use it. Resort to this power in difficult moments; use it to resist tempting foods that do not meet your nutritional needs. Abandon those foods that have no place in your diet. Everyone experiences moments of temptation. Strive toward strength and resistance; think success and banish thoughts of weakness and failure.

All these words sound fine and dandy until you come face to face with a favorite fattening food: a hot fudge sundae smothered with whipped cream, a delicious pie or cake à la mode, or a spicy, steaming sausage pizza. Are you sure the power to resist such foods is going to be present? The answer is YES! The power is present all the time. The reason it will work for you is simple: health overrides disease, goodness overrides evil, positive thinking overrides negative thinking, and truth overrides falsehood. This is the way of the Universe. Your body and mind are so uniquely and perfectly constructed that they continuously move in the direction of self-healing. You are going against Nature and the scheme of things if you become unhappy, fat and diseased. Health and wellbeing are the natural states of every form of life. Take a spiritual and physical approach to losing weight naturally and, without doubt, health will be yours.

BUT I'M HAPPY THE WAY I AM—FAT

Those who declare happiness despite carrying excess pounds are taking great risks with their health. Appetite may be properly said to be the beginning of disease, and if catered to, it usually leads only to increased craving. Overeating burdens the digestive and glandular systems and places a heavy tax on the excretory system. Excess food is bound to accumulate as waste and decompose into poisons. Certain diseases, such as diabetes, pneumonia, kidney disease, liver disease, high blood pressure, apoplexy and heart disease are more common in overweight than in thin or normal-weight people. Fat people may develop tumors and cancer out of their excess. Childbirth is more difficult for overweight women than for normal-weight women.

The accumulation of excess fat reduces the efficiency of every one of your body functions. Fat people, like fat animals, tend to be sterile. This fact was first observed more than two thousand years ago by Aristotle, who said: "Men and women who are fat are less prolific than those who are not fat," and "Fat animals have less seed than those that are lean."

The fat person is handicapped if an acute disease

develops. In pneumonia, for instance, the fat person has far less chance of survival. Fat individuals are often in generally poor physical condition. Wounds and operations heal more slowly for them than for other groups. Resistance to infection is generally lower than that of the normal person.

Fat is a great burden. It drags upon the spine, producing fatigue and backache. To resist the forward pull of an oversized front and maintain balance, the overweight man or woman must constantly lean backward from the hips. Thus, spinal muscles are maintained in a constant state of contraction and tension. The spinal column may become stiff, with an exaggerated forward curve of the small of the back, a condition known as lordosis.

Fat infiltrates the muscles, weakening them. When this takes place in the abdominal muscles, their normal support for the abdominal organs is crippled and the organs tend to sag or fall. Because of the weakening of the abdominal wall by fatty infiltration plus the constant presence of sagging organs, hernia is a common development. Rupture (hernia) in a heavy abdomen is a more serious condition than in a slender one and the seriousness increases as more weight is gained. Excess fat may surround and crowd the heart, rendering it less efficient. The overweight individual with high blood pressure overworks both heart and arteries. "Every pound of extra fat that is not normal to you contains 200 miles of extra capillaries," says Hygienist Dr. M. M. Bhamgara. Fat increases the amount of body volume through which the blood must be sent, thus causing blood pressure to rise. This may eventually result in degeneration of the kidneys and premature death.

You can hardly expect fat-oppressed digestive organs to function efficiently. This is especially true of those organs, like the stomach, whose function requires motion. They don't have room to move freely. In the very obese, there is considerable pressure not only on digestive organs but also on other vital organs. In the kidneys, this pressure narrows the passages of tubes and interferes with normal function. The overweight asthmatic finds not only his lungs but his whole body panting for more oxygen. Carrying ten to twenty pounds of excess weight also increases the joint pain suffered by an arthritic.

Fat is one of the chief causes of fallen intestine or colon, floating kidney, and malpositions of the womb. Fat also helps to produce varicose veins in the legs. There is no illness in which fat acts as an advantage to the body. The only possible benefit would be to someone stranded on an island for months without food. There is no period in life in which carrying excess weight is beneficial. Even fat infants have a higher death rate than those of normal weight if all other factors are equal. Obesity and health never coexist side by side.

There's no doubt about it. Being overweight is detrimental to your health. It is the primary reason for rejection for life insurance, exceeding the combined total of the four next most common reasons for rejection. Life insurance figures reveal that fat people do not often reach old age. The death rate after age forty is particularly high for obese persons. The suicide rate and number of fatal accidents is also high among fat men and women.

The following insurance figures, based on the definition of obesity, are significant:

Pounds Overweight	Percentage of Increased Mortality
10	8
20	18
30	28
40	48
50	58
60	61
70	81
80	116

From *Human Beauty, Its Culture and Hygiene* by Herbert M. Shelton

The whole truth about obesity is not commonly known, and the dangers of acquiring the habit of overeating at an early age are usually overlooked. Being overweight between the ages of twenty and thirty-nine may be serious, if the individual is twenty-eight to eighty pounds above average. Statistical studies reveal that if a man is twenty pounds overweight at forty-five, his chances of living to an old age are reduced by half. The body is said to begin breaking down gradually at middle age, and the excess load of fat hastens the breakdown process. After age sixty, the percentage of obese individuals in the population is less because many do not live beyond this age. Of course, some members of all weight groups die young and some heavyweights do live beyond sixty. There is still much to be learned about the relationship of weight to length of life. But while many factors help to determine length of life, fat definitely threatens longevity. Fat also adds to an uncomfortable life, to the development of disease, and to lowered working efficiency.

If you are happy in spite of being overweight, it

should be easier for you to begin a weight-loss program. Most happy people want to live as long as possible. To foster this, you must treat your body fairly, with kindness and respect. Why not reduce it to its most beautiful potential? It will perform better and last a lot longer.

CHAPTER TWO

THE DOS, THE MUSTS, THE IMPORTANT START

PROPER FOOD is not *even half of nutrition*. To be properly nourished means more than to eat natural foods in correct combinations. Equally important are healthy digestion and assimilation of food, and adequate disposal of waste. Many other factors also profoundly affect nutrition. A world of wisdom is contained in the biblical statement, "Man does not live by bread alone."

Water, oxygen and sunshine are also necessary nutritive materials. As activity, rest, sleep, warmth and your state of mind are vitally important to normal nutritive processes, building up the body, manufacturing secretions and eliminating waste matter from the blood and tissues are equally important. Growth, development, maintenance, repair and reproduction are all accomplished through nutritional materials. Therefore, in addition to a dietary program designed to promote weight loss, the following imperatives are important in order to supply all parts of your body with the needed nutritive materials. No one material is more important than any other.

RECEIVE *ALL* THE NUTRITIVE MATERIALS

Do Have an Exercise Program. It is a law of life that exercise influences nutrition and body function. Movement is life. Accounts of long-lived individuals commonly state that they were constantly active physically. And many of these individuals did much activity outdoors. Many people find they can endure nearly twice as much activity, exercise or work outside in the fresh air as they can indoors.

Being physically active means increased circulation. Circulation of blood and lymph constitutes the grand vital process by which food materials are floated to cells and tissues. Good circulation depends for its highest efficiency upon muscular activity, so exercise in some form becomes essential.

Many books on exercise can fit your needs. Read one or several. Have a varied exercise program that develops speed, endurance, flexibility and muscle coordination. Swimming, walking, bicycling, aerobic exercise and dance, skiing, skating and jogging are activities that involve both sides of the body and are highly worthwhile. Activities which emphasize one side of the body—tennis, baseball, bowling—are substantially less beneficial.

Avoid vigorous physical exercise after a heavy meal,

17

because the functions of the digestive organs are in high gear. If at the same time the skeletal muscles are required to perform strenuously, their withdrawal of blood from the digestive organs will greatly reduce or even suspend the digestive function. If you are going to be very active after a meal, either skip the meal entirely or eat lightly of easily digested foods.

More activity and less food, when the amount of surplus weight present is barely perceptible, will free your body of the threatened excess. More daily exercise is valuable both in preventing the accumulation of fat and in building up and maintaining normal vigor. Often a diet fails simply because the importance of stimulating the metabolism with a regular program of exercise has been overlooked. The man or woman who neglects this facet of life is sure to have his or her health and tissue condition deteriorate. Don't underestimate the role of activity in maintaining health and wellbeing.

Do Get Adequate Rest and Sleep. Rest and sleep are as important as exercise. Your alertness and entire wellbeing are hindered without adequate sleep. Alternate periods of activity and repose nourish the strength and regeneration of every organ. Sleep is necessary for the replenishment of exhausted nutrients in the cells. During sleep, the pulse rate decreases, skin vessels dilate, and blood pressure drops. Sleep rests the heart, equalizes the blood and restores the energy of the brain and nerve cells. The digestive system also rests during sleep. Food is best taken after and not before a period of sleep, for when you are tired, your digestive system will be proportionately unable to digest a meal.

Rather than taking a coffee break, take a relaxation

break. Without the use of a stimulant, it will be more beneficial in promoting your health and prolonging your life. If it is possible, a short period of rest in the middle of the day in a quiet, well-ventilated, darkened room is best. This does not mean actual sleep. Fifteen minutes with eyes closed in a horizontal position is more restorative than two hours sitting up. This will enable you to continue activities with greater ease than if no period of rest had been taken. Besides a short rest, complete changes of mental interests or scenery will also act as a re-energizer. Learn to know what your body needs. Don't go out to dinner or dancing when you clearly need a period of rest. Such continuous overtaxing and overworking your body may lead to a mental and physical breakdown.

Acquire the habit of spending a few minutes each day on the floor or on your bed relaxing your entire body. Start from your head and concentrate on each part of your body, relaxing each muscle in turn from scalp to toe. Produce a mental picture of what you want to be and what you will be. Love yourself enough to care.

Do Take Sunbaths. Sunshine's role in the nutritional processes is vital. Not just warmth and light, but the total rays of the sun are essential to full nutrition, full development and growth. Sunshine enables your body to manufacture vitamin D and makes it possible for you to utilize materials in the foods that build bones and teeth.

Ten minutes per day in the sun is a must. Taking a sunbath early in the morning or late in the afternoon or evening is better so as to avoid those ultra-hot rays in the middle of the day. Many people spend longer periods in the sun. Overexposure can be enervating, can age the skin and may also lead to skin cancer, especially if oils or creams are used. Learn your own limits. There is no arbitrary rule. What may be too much sun for one person may have no effect on another. In the winter months, if you can't get to a warm climate, sit at an open window, (next to a heater for warmth) and let the sun's rays shine on your body as the next best thing to being outdoors. And remember, the less clothing you have on, the better for receiving the sun's full benefit.

Do Avoid Extremely Hot or Cold Baths. A cold plunge or a short hot bath acts as a stimulant. You experience a brief feeling of wellbeing, an increase of physiological function, but this is always and necessarily followed by an equal amount of mental and physiological depression. Prolonged cold baths act much the same as does taking in harmful substances. The temporary exhilaration is soon followed by a decrease in function. Heart action is reduced, circulation and respiration slow down and nervous activity decreases. Muscular activity is decreased, even to the point of stopping. Prolonged application of cold to the chief trunk of a nerve will greatly diminish or entirely abolish its activity. The feeling of warmth that comes with the reaction from the first shock of the cold gives way to a feeling of chilliness and then cold. The apparent increase of strength gives way to a feeling of weakness and lassitude, and if the cold is continued, numbness and cessation of function follow. The initial feeling of increased strength from a cold plunge is actually the manifestation of vital resistance. Cold does not supply functional power; it causes its expenditure.

A hot bath dilates the arteries, capillaries, veins and lymph vessels. This temporarily increases skin activity. If the heating is prolonged or repeated often, the skin is weakened and its reactive power lessened; debility and exhaustion follow. Any prolonged or repeated stimulation, by whatever agent, always has this result.

Do Get Fresh Air. Respiration introduces oxygen into the body. Respiratory movements are important in assisting circulation of the blood. In "death" by drowning the victim is not resuscitated by working on the heart. Rather, artificial respiration is used to restore circulation and heart action.

Cell functions require a constant fresh supply of oxygen—the "master artist" in nature's workshop. Without fresh oxygen, every function of the body is lowered and the fluids and tissues of the body cannot be perfect.

CALORIES ARE BORING

Food values are frequently measured in calories. The calorie is a unit of measurement, just as the inch or yard is a unit of measurement. It is the amount of heat required to raise one kilogram (equal to about two and one-fourth pounds) of water one degree centigrade. It has been generally decided that the average male requires about 2,500 calories daily, the average female 2,000.

A table giving the caloric values of different foods tells you merely how much heat can be produced in the laboratory by burning these foods. This type of "firebox dietetics" implies that eating is simply a matter of supplying our system with food (calories or heat units) to produce energy. Heat and energy are considered equivalent and transformable.

Calorie tables are fairly accurate indexes to the heat and fuel values of the foods listed. They are not, however, an index to the food's nutritive values, such as mineral and vitamin content. You must digest, absorb, assimilate, and then metabolize these nutrients. If you fail to digest and absorb, you certainly cannot assimilate and metabolize.

You won't count calories on the diet in this book, because the caloric value includes only the combustible portion of a food. Your body is more than a mere furnace which you must fuel. The fuel value of food is really the least valuable thing about it. For example, white sugar is a very high-grade fuel, having a value of 1,750 calories per pound, as compared to 165 calories for buttermilk and 95 calories for spinach. Yet animals fed on white sugar and water will soon die. And eventually so will humans. A person will starve on such a diet while consuming more calories each day than the standard recommendations call for. He or she will die more quickly on this diet than if nothing but water is taken. The body adapts better to feeding upon its own balanced food reserves than on a prolonged diet of white sugar and water.

The nutritional value of foods can no more be measured in calories than the value of water in your body can be stated in pounds or quarts. Measuring food value by calories not only ignores the body's mineral and vitamin needs; it gives no attention to the protein value of a food. Proteins do not serve primarily as fuels in the body, but as building materials. Knowing the caloric value of a protein has nothing to do with its important amino acid content. Nor do calories assist in building bones and teeth.

A system of eating based on the caloric or fuel value of foods can cause the individual to be stuffed with fuel foods that are deficient in vital elements. No one should eat beyond their own particular digestive capacities in an effort to eat the "standard" amount of calories. There are no "standard" amounts of caloric needs, because each individual is unique. The amount of heat and energy required by various individuals differs greatly with temperament, occupation, age, size and sex. Aside from this, most of the heat produced by metabolizing food in the body is used in maintaining normal body temperature, not for the production of energy. If health is destroyed and if nutritive functions are impaired, stoking up on "fuel foods" is not only valueless, but positively harmful.

Counting calories is tiresome and boring. We believe that the sooner calorie counting is abandoned, the sooner normal weight can be obtained and maintained. Concentrate on the organic minerals and health-promoting factors contained in foods. Realize the importance of the digestive and assimilative powers of your body. Put your calculator away. Why not count happy moments instead?

WHAT ABOUT WEIGHING IN?

To weigh in or not to weigh in is a question that confronts most dieters. Often, you don't need to get on a scale to tell if you are overweight. If you *feel* fat, chances are you *are* fat. Rather than keep your eye on the scale, it is best to concentrate on how you feel about yourself. How you look, an awareness of the many good things you are doing for your body, and your state of mind are more important.

Frequent weighing is not advised. Getting on and off the scale each day may tell you, "Boy, look how easy it is to lose weight!" Making this wonderful discovery may cause you to go off the diet the next day. On the other hand, after getting off the scale, you may lament, "Woe is me! No diet ever works for me. What the heck, I'm so depressed I'll eat more food." Better to learn how to think positively. Science is realizing the vast powers of the mind. If you believe you will never lose weight, chances are you won't.

And what about those plateaus everybody reaches when dieting? It's not a good idea to weigh in frequently during the plateau period that often occurs after following a diet for three weeks. Our advice is to weigh yourself no more than once a week. Watch the mirror, and your thoughts, rather than the scale.

If people would eat only of the fruits of the trees there would be no plague.

LEONARDO DA VINCI (1452–1519)
Artist and scientist

CHAPTER THREE

DETERRENTS TO SUPERIOR NUTRITION

IN THIS CHAPTER we have listed alphabetically some of the items to avoid on your weight-loss program. Beverages to avoid are found in Chapter Four. A number of things deter superior nutrition, some more harmful to the body than others. The most detrimental are tobacco, alcohol, denatured foods, coffee and salt. Your persistent desire to change your former dietary habits is the key. Iron in your will is more important to nutrition than iron in your food.

Always praise yourself for avoiding harmful foods. Don't dwell on negative thinking. Don't set goals that are unrealistic. You're an okay person and humans have been known to slip occasionally. Learn to forgive yourself and start each day fresh. It is a rare person who can avoid all things that are unwholesome. But it must be understood that when certain items are damaging your nutrition, these must be corrected or eliminated. Only then can even the best of diets be properly utilized to the fullest.

Intelligent, reasoned observance of the laws of Nature is the only means of insuring perfect health.

ACIDOSIS OR HYPOALKALINITY

One of the most important deterrents to superior nutrition is a condition called acidosis or hypoalkalinity. The fluids of the body are normally slightly alkaline. Acidosis is the term misapplied to a lessened alkalinity of these fluids, a state more properly termed *hypoalkalinity*. Acidosis, or hypoalkalinity, is a condition characterized by a deficiency of fixed alkalies in the body, which leads to an increased production of ammonia in the urine and a high acidity.

Acidosis is not "acid blood," since the blood never becomes acid during life. An alkaline blood and lymph are necessary to life and health and for the blood to reach the point even of neutral pH would cause speedy death.

The normal ratio between the alkalies and acids of the body is approximately eighty to twenty—80 percent alkali and 20 percent acid. This proportion is maintained in balance by the so-called "buffer salts," sodium, potassium, calcium and magnesium, from which either side may draw as need arises. When this buffer or "balance wheel" is in normal order any excess of acids arising in the body is promptly neutralized. Only when there is a deficiency of buffer salts may troubles arise.

The body will not tolerate any free acid at all, except in the stomach during the process of digestion. All acids are instantly bound by being combined with alkalies to render them harmless. The body makes use of every resource at its command to preserve its alkalinity, because its cells can thrive only in an alkaline medium.

Since acids and alkalies are supplied by food, the matter of a balance between acid foods and alkaline foods is important. If you eat an excessive amount of acid food, your blood is forced to draw upon its alkaline reserve, its buffer salts, in order to maintain its normal alkalinity. When you have taken more acid than your body can bind without sacrificing some of the bases from the tissues, blood alkalinity falls below the normal level and you develop hypoalkalinity or acidosis.

Every food you eat leaves behind it an "ash" after it has been used by your body. The ash is either acid or alkaline. Eating too much acid-ash food, or eating it over long periods of time, results in storing acid ash in the cells and in depleting your body of its alkaline reserve.

A diet poor in alkaline foods, or eating food that has been robbed of its buffers has deleterious effects and contributes to a variety of serious diseases, such as arthritis and arteriosclerosis. Watch that the acids never predominate. Plan your meals with the following valuable acid-alkaline chart in mind, but don't make a fetish of it.

Other factors also affect normal alkalinity. Rest and sleep are alkalizers. So are exercise, fresh air, laughter, pleasure, conversation, enjoyment and love. Acidifiers are fear, anger, worry, gossip, hatred, envy, selfishness, silence and love-hunger. Always replace negative thoughts with positive thoughts and feelings.

Alkaline Fruits

apples
apricots
avocados
bananas (ripe)
berries (fresh)
cantaloupe
cherries
currants
dates
figs

grapes
grapefruit
lemons (use
  sparingly for
  flavor)
limes (use
  sparingly for
  flavor)
melons

nectarines
oranges
papayas
peaches
pears
pineapple (ripe)
raisins (organi-
  cally grown)
tangerines
tomatoes

Acidic Fruits

bananas
  (green) (NR)*
cranberries (NR)
olives
  (green) (NR)

plums
  (slightly acidic)
prunes
  (slightly acidic)

preserves, jellies
  and canned,
  sugared, dried,
  sulfured, or
  glazed fruits (NR)

*(NR) means not a recommended Hygienic food

Alkaline Vegetables

alfalfa sprouts
beans (string,
  lima, green)
beets
broccoli
cabbage
carrots
cauliflower
celery
chard
collards

cucumber
eggplant
endive
garlic (NR)
leek (NR)
lettuce
mung bean
  sprouts
mushrooms (NR)
  (non-digestible)

onions (NR)
parsley
parsnips
peppers (green
  and red)
potatoes
pumpkin
radish (NR)
spinach
squash
turnips

Acidic Vegetables

artichokes
asparagus tips
beans (dried)

brussels sprouts
garbanzos
  (chick-peas)

lentils
rhubarb (NR)

Alkaline Dairy Products

buttermilk (NR)   yogurt (home-   whey (NR)
                            made)
               raw milk (human, cow, goat)

Acidic Dairy Products

butter (unsalted)   cottage   ice cream (NR)
cheese   cheese (NR)   milk (other than
  (unprocessed)   raw) (NR)

Alkaline Meats

Acidic Meats

all meat, fish, fowl (NR)

Alkaline Nuts

almonds   chestnuts   coconut (fresh)
                            (roasted) (NR)

Acidic Nuts

all other nuts

Alkaline Cereals

corn (on the cob)   millet

Acidic Cereals

all refined boxed   corn (other than)   oats (rolled,
  cereals (NR)   on the cob;   unprocessed)
buckwheat   popcorn)   rice
  (unprocessed)   macaroni and   rye (unprocessed)
barley   spaghetti (NR) whole wheat
breads   noodles (NR)   bread
  (processed)(NR)   (unprocessed)

Other Acidic Foods

These foods are **not** *recommended*

alcoholic beverages	tea	egg whites
		horseradish
Coca-Cola and other soft drinks	cake candies	pastries
		spices
cocoa and chocolate	cookies dressings	sugar
		vinegar
coffee		yeast

WHAT TO AVOID

Every organ in the body, if not impaired or defective from birth or from causes occurring after birth, is capable of performing much more work than is necessary for the life of the organism. The muscular system, for instance, can greatly increase its work if it is called upon to do so. The kidneys are capable of increasing their activities and taking up part of the skin's work if, for any reason, the skin fails in its duties. The skin, when subjected to great heat or to vigorous muscular effort, can increase its cooling activities many times. The stomach, liver, intestines, bowels, heart or lungs are all capable of doing much more work than the actual needs of life require. The organs of a normal body can carry on the functions of life under all ordinary circumstances without strain, so long as they are not impaired by some cause or causes. The real challenge, therefore, is to find and remove the causes of organic impairment and deterioration.

Cells that are kept clean and properly nourished lose their vitality more slowly than cells that aren't. Certain organs and functions, when normal, completely rid the body of waste and toxins. Another process, when normal, keeps the cells freshly supplied with nutrient material. This nutrient material prevents the cells from rapidly growing old, from losing their vitality and dying too quickly.

Cells die by starvation and by poisoning. They are poisoned by excesses of food and by unnatural substances. They are starved when denatured foods that impair digestion and assimilation are eaten. To lose weight, to insure the efficiency of digestion and assimilation, and to help prevent premature aging, you should avoid, as much as possible, the following:

Animal Foods. This diet is a vegetarian program that includes unprocessed cheese, unsalted butter and raw milk. Vegans, or total vegetarians, do not eat dairy products.

Avoidance of flesh foods is nothing new. It has long been a part of the Hindu religion. Plato, Socrates, Ovid, Aristotle and Buddha were vegetarians, as were Leonardo, Tolstoy, Emerson and Thoreau.

In the late nineteenth century, British philosopher and playwright George Bernard Shaw stated, "A man of my spiritual intensity does not eat corpses." Nobel Prize-winning poet Rabindranath Tagore echoed this view at the turn of the twentieth century: "We manage to swallow flesh only because we do not think of the cruel and sinful thing we do." Shortly afterward, Indian nationalist leader Mahatma Gandhi said, "I hold flesh-food to be unsuited to our species. We err in copying the lower animal world if we are superior to it."

More recently, in 1973, author and biochemist Isaac

Asimov made the following prediction: "More and more in the next thirty years, we are going to be resorting to a vegetarian diet." And today we read such warnings from popular writers Gary and Steve Null: "The meat we eat may be killing us."

The high biological value of flesh proteins is not to be denied. However, we do not recommend their use. Flesh foods are merely mentioned in this program to give it a wider appeal. We understand that vegetarianism includes only a minority of people. But we condemn flesh-eating for these four reasons:

First: When flesh foods are eaten in large quantities, we take in more protein than we need. This produces harmful consequences. The average digestion can handle no more than four ounces of meat at a time without some putrefaction. Undigested protein may contribute to obesity, tumors, arthritis, premature aging, arteriosclerosis, nervous and mental disorders and a host of other ailments. Excess protein creates a general state of toxemic poisoning in the system, favoring the development of almost any illness.

Second: Meat contains considerable quantities of metabolic waste products, which are held up in the animal's tissues at the time of death. These wastes are poisonous. They are irritating and lend to meat a stimulating property that is usually mistaken for a quick pickup of added strength. The stimulation felt from eating meat stems from a high concentration of proteins and from the adrenalin which the animal secreted because of fear.

Third: Meat spoils easily. It is impossible to get it

before some degree of putrefaction has taken place. It further decays in the digestive tract. The poisons that form in your stomach and intestines are similar to those that form if the meat is allowed to decay in the refrigerator.

Fourth: The animals used for food consumption today are raised in animal factories, not on farms. Jim Mason and Peter Singer, in their book *Animal Factories,* vividly and dramatically portray the confinement practices and the mechanized systems designed to permit large-scale production with little labor.

Crowding masses of animals together causes stress, filth and other conditions that breed disease. To cope with these problems, farmers employ antibiotics, sulfa drugs, pesticides, disinfectants and a battery of other chemical products.

Food from animals raised in such an environment is not only of poor quality but can also contain chemical residues dangerous to humans.

Condiments. Condiments are in almost universal use. Many condiments are regarded as a natural and necessary part of the diet, but they actually improve the palatability of foods only for those who are accustomed to their use. No condiment is palatable when it is first tasted. Everyone is forced to learn to use them over the protest of his/her organic instincts. Using condiments is really a deliberately cultivated perversion of the sense of taste. The addition of condiments, sauces, seasonings, salt and pepper, spices, vinegar and so forth, camouflages the fine, delicate flavors that Nature put into food products and prevents the user from enjoying them fully. Always keep in mind that condiments irritate the mucous membranes which line all the internal organs. They cause inflammation, induration (thickening) and ulceration and can be a contributing factor in cancer.

Losing weight and using condiments do not go well together, because condiments increase your appetite. The desire for food should arise out of actual physiological needs and, when these natural needs are not present, no food should be eaten. Stimulating your appetite by the use of condiments leads to overeating. So great is the power of condiments to stimulate appetite that it is almost impossible to overeat if they are *not* employed. Compare the number of people who overeat pineapples to the number who overeat pasta or enchiladas.

The overeater's disturbed appetite is sometimes caused by acquiring a taste for certain condiments. The taste enslaves its victims. In chlorosis (a form of anemia), pregnancy and certain mental and nervous ailments, patients often crave the most singular and disgusting articles. Disturbed or inadequate nutrition may be at the foot of much of this perversion. A lack of minerals or vitamins can give rise to a vague, ill-defined craving that causes the patient to eat anything in an effort to satisfy it. But abnormal cravings often disappear when the use of stimulants is discontinued.*

There are other reasons why people should stop using stimulating condiments. They do not supply any nutritional need in the body and all of them are harmful. Condiments irritate the digestive organs and im-

*This topic is discussed in detail in *Fasting for the Health of It* by H. M. Shelton and Jean A. Oswald.

pair and depress their function. They blunt the sensibilities of the gustatory nerves and thereby diminish the enjoyment of simple foods. Mustard, pepper, horseradish, spices, cloves, ginger, nutmeg, etc., differ only in the degree of their irritating qualities. They all exert their irritating effect upon the delicate membranes of the digestive tract; they excite the stomach to increased action in certain respects but lessen the secretion of gastric juice and, later, decrease stomach activity. Repeated irritation from these substances produces irreparable injury to the stomach, liver, intestine, kidneys, blood vessels, heart and other vital organs. Catarrh (inflammation of a mucous membrane, especially of the nose or throat), chronic inflammation, glandular destruction, permanently impaired digestion, gastric ulcer, cancer of the alimentary canal and colitis are among the results of using condiments.

Few people completely abandon condiments. Advising a person not to use condiments is like asking a person not to get wet while standing in the rain. Many will use substitutes, coffee substitutes, candy substitutes and "health" condiments if asked to abandon the originals. Anise seed, celery and caraway seed, sage, paprika, nutmeg—the less irritating substances—will replace cayenne, mustard, horseradish and other hot and exciting substances. Celery salt and various other vegetable salts (which are made up largely of common salt) still will be employed. Although these things are not as bad as some of the substances they replace, dieters and health-seekers should know that they still disguise the natural flavors of food, act as irritants, and induce overeating.

Denatured Foods. Denatured foods are foods that have been altered and impaired in the process of manufacturing by bleaching, canning, cooking, preserving, refining, frying, baking, boiling, diluting, separating, emulsifying and/or pickling. Foods that have undergone these processes before being sold are no longer as well fitted to meet the needs of the body as they were in the state in which Nature prepared them.

All this does not mean that you eat a diet of 100 percent raw foods. Obviously some vegetables and grains need to be cooked to be edible. The ideal ratio is 80 percent raw fruits and vegetables and 20 percent cooked.

Except for fresh fruits and vegetables, practically everything has had something done to it. Milk is pasteurized, condensed, evaporated or boiled; eggs are from hens that lay two or three hundred a year and are fed on "rich" fare that produces disease in them. Sugar is crystallized, refined and bleached. As a result, the sap of cane or beet has had all the minerals and vitamins removed from it. Cereals are cracked, rolled, flaked, roasted, boiled and "shot from cannons." Wheat is milled, removing its minerals and vitamins,and the flour is bleached and chemicalized. The most important food elements are removed in the milling process. Flesh foods are smoked, pickled, salted, canned, sausaged, refrigerated, and kept for long periods before being eaten. Dried fruits are heated in drying, bleached with sulfur dioxide, stored for long periods of time, and finally stewed and mixed with white sugar before being eaten.

Is all this good for us? No way! The processes to which foods are subjected destroy the highly delicate

::::::::::::::::::::::::::::

and tender vital food factors. A nation whose diet is made up almost wholly of denatured foods cannot possibly be well nourished.

Some people may think they can eat larger amounts of fresh fruits and vegetables along with the denatured foods and then everything will be all right. That is not the case. It's like taking an antidote when you take a poison. Instead, stop taking the poison. Offsetting denatured foods with large quantities of fresh fruits and vegetables entails a hardship upon the organs of digestion and elimination. And even if the diet is half denatured and half natural, the natural foods will not be sufficient to compensate for the deficiencies in the denatured half.

Denatured foods will not sufficiently nourish the body, nor will they build good bones and nerves or normal blood. On a diet consisting of a single denatured food or combination of foods, animals die.

Dr. Roger J. Williams, in his book *Nutrition Against Disease*, shows how personalities can actually change after eliminating denatured foods and replacing them with more nutritious foods.

According to a London study, seventeen delinquent girls, eleven to fifteen years of age, had been on a diet made up largely of white bread and margarine, cheap jam, lots of sweet tea, and canned and processed meats. When their diet was changed to one that was far more nutritious and diversified, not only did their complexions and physical wellbeing improve "almost beyond recognition," but they quickly became less aggressive and quarrelsome. Bad habits seemed to disappear; the "problem children" became less of a problem, and the bored ones began to take an interest in life.

You can't expect a healthy, productive life if you wake yourself up with caffeine, eat a denatured diet, incorrectly combine your foods, coax your appetite with condiments, forget about exercising, neglect to get fresh air and sunshine, and then go to sleep with the aid of a barbiturate. Don't question the fact that your energy level is low and you often have a listless feeling. Now you have the answer.

Dried Beans. Beans such as kidney beans, pinto beans and navy beans contain about 25 percent protein and approximately 50 percent carbohydrate or starch. Each of their two principal constituents requires entirely different processes for digestion. The strong gastric juice of the stomach, which is engaged in digesting proteins, impedes starch digestion. This undoubtedly accounts for the difficulty in digesting beans and the readiness with which they ferment. Except under the most favorable circumstances, these ferments produce gas and toxins.

One of the best rules is to eat as few beans as possible, with the exception of green or yellow beans and limas. These contain less starch than the matured or dried beans that produce gas. The philosopher and mathematician Pythagoras advised that we eat no beans. Hygienists subscribe to that tenet, making an exception only in the case of beans that contain little starch.

Egg Whites. Eggs have about the same protein composition as the human body. A young pig may gain a pound a day, but a child rarely gains an ounce a day. In fact, it sometimes takes a child fifteen years to gain one hundred pounds. If for fifteen years a child ate only the protein contained in one egg a day, the child would have eaten six times the protein equivalent of her own body. On the plan of rearing children on one or two pounds of meat, milk, eggs, legumes, cheese and bread a day, the growing child passes through his liver and kidneys enough protein to build two to four thousand pounds of human flesh. This is a needless strain on the body.

The more closely a food resembles the human body in composition, the more its consumption in large amounts becomes harmful. Flesh foods are the worst offenders, eggs come second and milk is next.

Eggs at best are poor foods. Modern methods of egg production, involving great overstimulation of laying, produce eggs of very poor quality.

The unfitness of certain foods for assimilative purposes is made evident by symptoms that so frequently follow their use.

Raw egg white is poorly digested and assimilated. From 30 to 50 percent of the egg white consumed passes through the digestive canal without being digested and absorbed. Raw egg white may produce diarrhea and sometimes vomiting. Egg whites (raw or cooked) are acid-forming and produce almost deadly acids in some stomachs. Practically all constipated people are sensitive to white of egg poisoning. Invalids, inactive people, overweight people and those inclined to constipation especially should avoid egg whites. They are also bad food for children and for those whose liver or kidneys are not in perfect condition.

Numerous experiments have shown that:

1. Egg white (raw or cooked) hinders the action of the digestive fluids.

2. Egg white contains a poison which may damage the kidneys (avidin, a biotin-inactivating protein).

The habit of eating whole eggs can cause constipation, obesity, headaches, asthma, epilepsy, arthritis, high blood pressure and high blood cholesterol.* Eating just the yolk of the egg is less objectionable. The yolk is an alkaline-ash food, but the white is an acid-ash food. Egg yolks are easily digested and, if eaten raw in small amounts with a green salad, are not the source of any trouble. They should be from fertile eggs.

Honey. Honey may be classified as an animal food. The true vegetarian does not eat it. The fact that honey is classed as a *laxative* and as a diuretic indicates its unfitness for human use. Fruit sugar is superior to honey as a human nutrient. The value of honey is ludicrously lauded in many quarters. Honey, when compared with the fruit sugars, ranks about on the level with white sugar.

Honey serves the needs of the bees, but is of little nutritional value to humans. Honey is a poor source of nutrients other than sugar, being devoid of protein, exceedingly poor in minerals and possessing almost no vitamins. Honey contains formic acid, which diminishes its digestibility. Due to this preservative, it will keep for several years. Honey will ferment, however, and bees have been known to get drunk on fermented honey. It is sad to note that many beekeepers now feed the bees stale candies from candy factories.

Honey also often contains bacteria that cause botulism, a disease particularly dangerous to infants aged

*Consult Dr. Shelton's *Hygiene System,* Volume 2 (1935) for more about this topic.

nine months or younger, who therefore should never be fed honey. *(U.S. Pharmacist,* 9 #5:21, 1984). Symptoms range from bloating, constipation and general weakness to paralysis and respiratory depression because of weakness of the diaphragm and chest muscles. The toxin produced by botulism bacteria causes relaxation of all muscles. It also has been conjectured that botulism may be responsible for many cases of sudden infant death (crib death).

Salt. Salt is a powerful irritant. The sharp pain that comes from placing a single grain of salt into the eye or a cut reveals its irritating power. Taken into the body, it has the same irritating effect upon the internal tissues and nerves.

Common salt is a poison. In some sections of China, people commit suicide by drinking a pint of a saturated solution of common salt. Its powerful laxative effect is further evidence that salt is a poison. The increased bowel action is the body's means of expelling the unwanted salt from the digestive tract. An infant can die from an enema of 1:16 salt solution. Whether salt is diluted in a solution or sprinkled on a potato, it is nevertheless a poison.

An accumulated ounce of salt in the tissues requires about three quarts of water to hold it in solution. If you have four ounces of salt in your system, you will carry about three gallons of water in your body. This would add close to twenty-four pounds of body weight.

If a substance cannot be transformed into tissue, or if it cannot be used in the production of secretions, its use is unnecessary.

Salt is eliminated with difficulty when it is in the

bloodstream. Much of it is thrown out through the skin. Indeed most of the solid matter in sweat is sodium chloride. The perspiration of heavy salt users is more like brine than anything else. When this dries on clothes, sufficient salt is often left on them to streak them with white lines and blotches. The tears of salt eaters are also salty, while the tears of the non-user are not. Overly salt tears are irritating to the eyes. Isn't it reasonable that since Nature's purpose for tears is to lubricate and cleanse the eyes, tears should not be irritating to them?

It is a fallacy to believe that the use of salt is instinctive. Mineral elements cannot be taken into the body in their crude state and used. Salt is no exception to this rule. It is both indigestible and unassimilable. Salt enters the body as a crude, inorganic substance; it is absorbed from the intestine unchanged and goes the rounds of the general circulation unassimilated. It is finally eliminated from the body in the same state it entered.

Students of Thoreau will recall that he abandoned the use of salt after he discovered that the Indians did not use it. They maintained a high standard of health and physical efficiency without salt. Also in literature, Robinson Crusoe's Friday did not use salt. Numerous people have not used it. In fact, the greater part of the human race has lived and died without ever knowing of its existence. A careful study of the history of our own European and American people will reveal that the general use of salt is a rather recent custom. This modern custom should be abandoned. Salts should be obtained from unprocessed, unrefined, natural foods.

The salt-eating habit is all part of "the white plague"

(salt, white flour and refined sugar) that is overtaking our supermarket shelves. According to Hygienist Frank D. Sabatino, D.C., health depends on a well-regulated balance of fluid and charged particles (electrolytes) between the interior of body cells and the surrounding extracellular sea in which they float. In his article "The White Plague" in *Hygienic Review,* July 1979, he says, "Though the entire electrolyte and mineral environment of the body is important, it is the movement and the relationship of sodium to potassium that plays a primary role in the electrical dynamics and fluid balance at the level of the cell. Excess sodium irritates the delicate mucous membranes of the body and upsets the electrical balance of nerve cells. This can interfere with the normal transmission of impulses in our nervous system and can result in myriad varieties of cellular degeneration and organ dysfunction." Salt intoxication can start with simple edema and can progress through the destruction of cellular identity seen in arthritis, cancer and other end-point degenerative changes.

Because salt retards digestion, impairs the ability to absorb vitamins, changes blood chemistry, paralyzes the inner lining of the blood vessels, stimulates the heart, retards kidney function, paralyzes the secretory activities and is wholly unnutritious, you would do well to think twice before you say, "Please pass the salt"; said more accurately, it is "Please pass the poison."

Saturated Fried Fats. The fatty acids of fruits, nuts and other vegetable sources belong to a group of fats described as *polyunsaturated.* Two striking exceptions to this rule for vegetable fats are the oils of chocolate and the coconut. The fats of butter, milk, lard and other animal fats are heavily *saturated*. The saturated fats are accused of being partly responsible for high blood cholesterol, atherosclerosis, high blood pressure and heart disease. The oils of nuts, the avocado, sunflower seeds, peanuts, the soybean and grains are much better adapted to human use than the fats of beef, lamb, pork and dairy products.

Hygienists emphasize that prolonged heating of fatty foods, as in baking or frying, destroys some of their essential fatty acids. In oils or butter used for frying, fats tend to be rancid. This is but one of the reasons to refrain from eating fried foods.

Ohio State University cancer researcher John P. Minton substantiates the Hygienic view by claiming that the cooking oils used by fast-food restaurants may be linked to an increase in the rate of stomach cancer.

(A 1983 article *Milwaukee Journal* April 3,1983) titled "Rise in Stomach Cancer Linked to Cooking Oils" supports his theory:

> John P.Minton said the incidence of stomach cancer in the United States, which had been declining for nearly eighty years, began increasing in the late 1970s. He suspects the fats in the often hastily assembled American diet.
>
> Minton said attention should be focused on oils used in fast-food restaurants, particularly when these oils were reheated.
>
> Scientists know that each time oil is heated its molecules break down a little more, Minton said. When the oil is eaten, it leads to an increase in unstable molecules in the body, which can create genetic cell injury, he said.

He said chemical changes in the oil, and the fat itself promoted cell division, making it easier for cancer cells to multiply and trigger a shutdown in the body's immune mechanisms.

Minton estimated that a change in the body that promoted cancer development could take twenty years.

Thus, Minton arrived at a "speculative concern" that the fast-food industry, which began its growth spurt in the mid-to-late 1950s, might have something to do with the increase in stomach cancer.

Minton said the highest incidence of stomach cancer in the world was in Japan, where people eat a lot of tempura, a food dipped in a batter and deep-fried in oil. In Japanese coastal areas, where residents are poorer and less inclined to discard their used oil, the stomach cancer rate is higher than in Tokyo.

Tars.

Tar is thick brown to black liquid consisting of a mixture of hydrocarbons and their derivatives obtained by the destructive distillation of many kinds of carbonaceous matter.

GOULD MEDICAL DICTIONARY

Tars are substances to avoid. Food that is subjected to great heat, as in frying, roasting or toasting undergoes decomposition, with the formation of highly complex black tar. Most people are familiar with the tar formed when tobacco is burned in a pipe. The bowl of the pipe and the pipestem become clogged with the sticky, foul-smelling stuff.

Tar forms in coffee while it is being roasted; it forms in cereals, beans and fruits when these are roasted to make coffee substitutes. Coffee drinkers and drinkers of coffee substitutes daily take tar into their bodies, just as the smoker gets tar into his mouth, throat, lungs and blood.

If potatoes, beans, peas or other vegetables become dry in cooking and get scorched, tar forms. Scorched toast has tar in it. In frying potatoes, eggs, meat and other foods, tar is often formed unless great care is exercised not to overheat these foods. Meats roasted in an oven that is too hot get black on the outside—tar is formed.

Tar is an irritant. It is one of the irritants that is known to result in the formation of tumors and cancers. It would be valuable to know the percentage of the tumors and cancers that exist today because of tars. Almost everyone eats cooked foods and drinks coffee or coffee substitutes. Breathing the air of smoggy cities also takes tar into the lungs. This, as much as tobacco smoke, may contribute to the production of lung cancer.

Tobacco. Nicotine is among the most deadly of poisons. If the skin of a mouse is pricked with a needle point that has been dipped in the essential oil of tobacco, the skin swells and the mouse dies. Introduce a piece of chewing tobacco the size of a kidney bean into the mouth of a robust man or woman unaccustomed to tobacco, and the skin pales, a cold sweat develops, the pulse flutters. Soon each will be affected with fainting, dizziness, nausea and vomiting. Such are a few of the effects of nicotine.

When tobacco is chewed, juice and tobacco particles are carried into the throat and swallowed. Reaching the stomach, they cause nausea at the time and indigestion later. Tobacco juice from cigars held in the mouth also finds its way to the stomach. During smoking, tobacco smoke enters the lungs and the nicotine is absorbed over a wide expanse of sensitive membrane. Both chewing and smoking tobacco greatly impair the senses of smell and taste. Even the nonsmoker in the room with a smoker is affected by tobacco fumes in the air; the younger the person or pet sitting in the room, the more easily their tissues are injured by the nicotine they are forced to inhale.

The first effect of stimulation from a substance such as tobacco is exaltation of physiological function; if the stimulation is long continued or often repeated, exhaustion with an almost total abolition of function results. The repeated use of stimulants would soon result in death if the organism had no means of curbing its own reactions and lessening the expenditure of vital power. But repeated stimulation soon brings about a condition in which the organism ceases to respond so readily and violently to the stimulant. If the former degree of stimulation is to continue to be received from a stimulant used repeatedly, a larger amount of the stimulant must be used each time.

The first smoke or the first chew of tobacco usually occasions a powerful reaction against it on the part of the organism. So long as the body's physiological powers and instincts are not habituated or impaired, they instantly perceive the poisonous character of the tobacco and give the alarm to the whole system. A vigorous effort is made to destroy and eliminate the invader, and the user is forced to throw away his tobacco. But if he continues to try tobacco, the reaction against it grows less and less with each repetition until, finally, a

smoker is able to use many times the original amount
without producing such violent results. The smoker's
body learns to tolerate the tobacco and adapts itself to
its use as far as possible. The system's natural re-
sponses soon become perverted; tobacco's poisonous
character is no longer detected and no alarm is given.
Instead, a craving for the substance develops. However, the habitual use of any substance that is injurious in itself will not ever render that substance harmless
or beneficial. The habitual presence of any such substance in the body is injurious to cell life, even though
the body's energetic efforts to resist its action may cease.

What is here said of tobacco is also true of other
poisonous substances. Frequently, a user of drugs such
as tobacco, opium, alcohol, cocaine, etc., becomes so
accustomed to them that he or she is able to take at one
time enough of the favorite drug to kill several nonus-
ers outright.

Everyone knows that smoking destroys the cells in
the body, contributes to the aging process, and is a
cause of disease. Smoking is one of the worst habits
that needlessly expend the body's vital energies.

Vinegar. Vinegar is that little unnecessary extra. Vinegar's highly toxic acetic acid content destroys ptyalin
(the salivary enzyme that converts starch into sugar).
Experiments have shown that as small a portion of
vinegar as one in 5,000 appreciably diminishes the
digestion of starch. One part in 1,000 renders starch
digestion very slow, and one part in 500 arrests it
altogether. From these facts it becomes evident that
vinegar, pickles (saturated with vinegar), salads on
which vinegar has been sprinkled and salad dressings
containing vinegar are unwholesome substances. This

is especially true when vinegar is eaten with starchy foods such as cereals, bread, legumes or potatoes.

Vinegar also contains alcohol, which precipitates the pepsin of the gastric juice and retards or prevents gastric digestion of proteins. Thus pickles and vinegar cripple the first stages of digestion of both starch and protein. Apple cider vinegar contains the same two virulent poisons, alcohol and acetic acid, so its use also impairs digestion.

Anything that inhibits the secretion of the digestive juices, alters their chemistry or destroys their enzymes will retard or suspend the process of digestion. Such foods are common causes of indigestion. There seems to be no good reason why you should eat foods at the same meal that either directly or indirectly interfere with each other's digestion.

THE PRINCIPLE OF THE HYGIENIC DIET

The principle of this diet is a simple one: whatever is foreign to a natural, healthy organism and cannot be digested and assimilated to its essential structure is obviously not capable of being processed by normal metabolic activities. These substances are inimical to your body and will cause weight gain, disease or both. Conforming to this principle, all substances that are nonusable by your body create a normal response of disrelish. Your senses of taste and smell will alert you. Nothing reveals more effectively the fitness of natural food for healthy life than the higher offices of taste and smell. When you bring unnatural substances into your stomach, confusion and upset reign. Respond to your body's signals, eat moderately from Nature's bountiful table, and you'll never be fat again.

A diet well-ordered bears the greatest prolongation of life.
FRANCIS BACON (1561–1626)
English philosopher

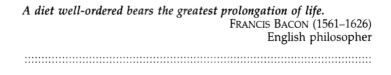

FACTS ABOUT BEVERAGES

IT'S EASY TO DRINK too much liquid. When tissues are overfilled with fluid, flabbiness takes the place of firmness and the aging process progresses more quickly. Whether you drink fruit or vegetable juices, teas, beer or just plain water, the result is the same—too much fluid.

Josiah Oldfield, M.D., a fruitarian from England, has examined desert Arabs and found them to be handsome and agile at an extreme old age. Oldfield says, "In spite of heat, dust, and exhausting fatigue, these desert wanderers drink but little, and at long intervals, and so retain physique and complexion to extreme old age." He adds that "Such Arabs drink less in a month than many a young English man or woman takes in a week."*

"When in India," said Dr. Oldfield, "I was horrified

*Herbert A. Shelton, *Human Beauty, Its Culture and Hygiene.*

by the rapidity with which charming, beautiful English women went off and lost color, softness of skin, and the vivacity of youth—largely owing to developing the habit of eternally drinking all day long, drinks of all sorts from tea and lemonades to pegs and cocktails." Water and sugar were the main constituents of these drinks. All of the changes observed by Dr. Oldfield cannot be attributed to fluid intake alone, but the excess liquids certainly accounted for some of them.

THE NUMBER ONE DRINK—WATER

Pure water is the best drink. All other fluids are either foods or poisons. The body contains an average of 70 percent water. Because water is being constantly lost through the lungs as vapor, through the skin as sweat and through the kidneys as urine, you have a need to replenish your water supply regularly. An average person excretes over three quarts of water a day.

Crystal-clean water helps you to retain youthfulness, but only if it is not taken excessively. The advice to drink lots of water to "flush" the system is absurd. Water has no such flushing effect. Lots of water does not increase elimination of waste—there is only an increased elimination of water.

Water supports all of the nutritive processes from digestion on through absorption and circulation—assimilation and disassimilation—to excretion. Some of the most important functions of water in the body are:

1. Water is an essential constituent of all tissues, cells and body fluids.

2. Water holds the nutritive materials in solution and

serves as a medium for the transportation of food to the various parts of the body.

3. Water holds waste and toxins in solution and serves as a medium for transportation of these out of the body.

4. Water keeps the various mucous membranes soft and prevents friction of their surfaces.

5. Water is used in regulating body temperature.

Water needs vary with age, sex, climate and activity. A person engaging in active physical labor in the summer sun requires more water than an office worker. You require more water in summer than in winter, more for the day's activities than during the night. The more food you eat, the more water your system will demand. The fasting individual has little thirst. A person whose diet is chiefly fruits and vegetables gets large quantities of water in its purest form. Most green vegetables and fresh fruits contain a higher percentage of water than do cells of the adult body. If your diet contains an abundance of these foods, little or no additional water will be required. More water is needed on a diet that consists of flesh or denatured foods.

If a sufficient amount of water is forced into a human or animal, it will produce all the symptoms of alcoholic intoxication. Nothing is gained by excess of any kind. Excessive water-drinking waterlogs tissues and lessens cell vitality. The power of the blood to absorb and carry oxygen is lowered and the body is weakened.

Observations and experiments demonstrate that people, animals and plant life are all injured by too much water. Supersaturation of the protoplasm of plants submerged in water weakens and even kills them. Excess

water produces rank, watery vegetation, while prolonged standing in water will kill most vegetation more
surely than a drought.

Hygienist Keki R. Sidhwa, D.O., D.C. says in an
article entitled, "Water-logged Tissues" in *Dr.
Shelton's Hygienic Review* for September 1964: "A cell overfull and
distended cannot work so energetically as one with its
proper amount of fluid, and a water-logged cell is in a
condition which renders it liable to be less efficient
than a normally constituted, virile cell. Where a cell
has its minimum supply of fluid its vitality is concentrated and its resistance to inimical influences is very
high."

You perspire more when drinking more, and excessive perspiring is also weakening. Generally those who
suffer most from the summer's heat are the people
who drink the most water. It's not that they drink
more because the heat causes great thirst. If these
individuals would drink less, their sweating would
decrease. The excessive drinking is largely responsible
for the sweating.

A slight excess of water is not particularly harmful.
The safest rule about drinking is: drink as little as thirst
demands. A false thirst induced by salt or some other
irritant is not to be "satisfied." Eating salty, spicy or
greasy dishes, concentrated foods, meats, eggs, or cheese
can also create an irritation that is mistaken for thirst,
but water will not relieve such a "thirst."

And don't drink a certain number of glasses of water
a day just because somebody has arbitrarily decided
that people "require" that much water. There is no
sound reason why water should be taken in the absence of real physiological need.

Water drinking can become a habit like any other. People who cultivate drinking large quantities of water will feel a "need" for much water. You can inundate your stomach with water every five minutes and still be "thirsty." If you refrain from drinking, this almost irresistible desire for water will pass away. On the other hand, if water is taken, natural secretions will not be used by your body to relieve the "thirst."

The Hygienic maxim of "drink only when you are thirsty" holds as true in 1985 as it did in 1850. Pioneer Hygienist Sylvester Graham particularly advised not to drink with meals. Animals in nature do not drink with meals. Grooms know enough to water their horses first and then, after an interval of time, feed them. Drinking with meals and directly after meals leads to dilation of the stomach, chronic indigestion, gastritis and ulcers.

Water first dilutes the digestive juices and their enzymes. Then it passes out of the stomach in five minutes and carries along with it the digestive juices and enzymes that it holds in solution. Even to drink two hours after meals is not always wise. It can mean flooding the stomach with water at the very time that the digestive juices are present in greatest abundance and the work of digestion is proceeding with the greatest efficiency. Also, the natural secretions found in the stomach prevent putrefaction and fermentation in the digestive tract, while water favors those very processes.

Unless irritating spices, salt or greasy dishes have been taken in the evening meal, you will have no need to drink water during the night. Nature is entirely competent in satisfying all needs if natural laws are not violated. Don't confuse *fictional* thirst and *genuine* thirst.

::::::::::::::::::::::::::::::

Alcohol. Alcohol, which for a very brief moment seems to strengthen and increase function, actually results in diminished function and weakness. Alcohol does not add power to your system. It only occasions the expenditure of power you already have. It is properly classed as a caustic irritant, and the enhanced functioning felt just after its intake is not due to any power it communicates to the body and mind, but rather to the body's resistance and consequent expenditure of vital power in reaction to the alcohol's irritating effects. The depression which follows is due to the exhaustion of vital powers and alcohol's destructive effects upon the tissues of the body.

Alcoholic beverages are classified as foods, but they are lethal to every cell in the body. Alcohol is a drug and a poison. It accelerates the aging process. Alcoholic beverages do not favor digestion. Wine interferes with salivary digestion of food and also retards digestion in the stomach. Wine, beer and other alcoholic beverages destroy pepsin, thus making gastric digestion impossible. Continued use impairs the body's efficiency in digesting and assimilating food, which later may result in cirrhosis of the liver, diabetes, hypoglycemia, nervous and mental disorders, or heart and kidney disease.

The excitement (*stimulation*) and increased temperature (*fever*) associated with the presence of alcohol in the body does not represent the same activity you have when you eat.

Alcohol not only expends energy, but also prevents the evolvement of energy. Its use squanders a person's functional resources and alienates those that would otherwise be re-energizing. Alcohol interferes directly with the nutritive processes through which alone the resources of life are converted into energy. It devitalizes all vital tissues.

Coffee, Tea and Carbonation. Coffee, whether caffeinated or decaffeinated, is harmful. Decaffeinated coffee is still a toxic beverage that the kidneys have to work hard to eliminate. Both types of coffee irritate the lining of the stomach. Regular coffee with caffeine is a stimulant (irritant) and makes unnecessary work for the heart. Author Joy Gross has this to say about coffee in her book *Thin Again: Improved Fitness in 30 Days:*

> Coffee has a pyridine base. The breakdown product of this chemical in your body is urea, the same toxic residue you get when you eat meat. Charles Eliot Perkins, a biochemist who's done extensive research in cancer, has found that the one substance that's common to all cancer-producing chemical compounds, without which there can be no cancer activity, is pyridine. It's the same chemical that's found in coal-tar, soot, and tobacco smoke.

Without doubt, coffee has no place in a wholesome diet. Neither does tea. Like coffee, it is a stimulant. Not only does it contain caffeine, but it contains tannic acid, which also acts as a diuretic. Juniper berry tea, mint tea, alfalfa tea, mistletoe tea, sassafras tea, parsley tea, strawberry tea and other teas increase the flow of urine. All this means is that they act as stimulants; the kidneys are forced to expel the tea quickly.

People who use noncaloric carbonated beverages will have less success on this weight-loss program. These drinks are loaded with sodium. When you eat nothing but natural foods for a significant period of time, you will develop a distaste for the artificial sweeteners found in diet beverages and soon won't want to drink them. Instead, about half an hour before a meal, drink a tall glass of water. Sip it slowly and you will discover that it will take the edge off a hearty appetite.

Fruit and Vegetable Juices. The habit of drinking juices— orange, grapefruit, tomato and celery, papaya—between meals is responsible for a large amount of indigestion in those who think they are eating healthfully. Drinking juices *is* eating. To drink them between meals inter- feres with digesting the previous meal, and trouble is sure to follow. Since the misuse or overuse of juices disorganizes digestion, our rule is: *Do not drink fruit and/or vegetable juices between meals.*

If you choose to include juices in your diet, have them one-half hour before your meal. The juice should properly combine with the meal. Or have the juice *as* the meal—such as a large orange-pineapple drink or a blended salad. Do keep in mind, however, when drink- ing juices or preparing a salad in a blender, that these will not give you the same nutritive value you would have from eating the foods whole.

MOTHER'S MILK IS FOR INFANTS

History shows us that a man by the name of Under- wood is apparently the first to have fed cow's milk to infants. This was in 1793. Prior to that date, if a mother died and left her child to be nursed, this was done by a wet nurse and not by the cow. Since then, the cow has become almost a foster mother in America. Cow's milk has been proclaimed as the "perfect food." It is recommended for the infant, the child, the athlete, the office worker, the invalid and everyone else. There is a strong commercial influence behind the magical virtues of milk. Despite the claims made by profiteers, cow's milk is constituted to meet best the requirements of a growing calf, not a growing child.

It is unnatural for cows to give the large quantities of milk, rich in fat, that our dairy cows do. By selective breeding and forced feeding, they are induced to give unusual quantities of milk and to produce far beyond the normal nursing period. Indeed, many of these cows are never "dry." They continue to produce milk that is sold in the market from one calf to the next, year after year. Cows have been observed to milk for ten or more years without once being dry, birthing one calf every twelve months. This constitutes a drain on the cows which makes it nearly impossible for them to be healthy. Dairy cows are especially prone to tuberculosis, and have greatly shortened lives.

Added to the evils of excessive milk production is the evil of overfeeding on a one-sided and high-protein diet. This tends to produce disease in the cow and greatly distorts the content of her milk. A diet high in protein causes putrefaction in the lactating mother. Combine this extra protein added to the diet of the cow with the fact that cow's milk naturally contains far more protein than that of a human mother anyway, and the effects on the human child are obvious. A slender, supple and fairly strong baby can become a logy, stiff, obese baby. Of the chubby babies so much admired, pioneer Hygienist Charles Page, M.D. (1840–1925), said:

"The excessive fat, so generally regarded as a sign of a healthy baby, is as truly a state of actual disease as when it occurs at adult age. Not only are the muscles enveloped with fat—they are mixed with it throughout and so are the vital organs—the kidneys, liver, heart, etc. Fat babies often present an appearance of dullness which is quite a contrast to the appearance and action of healthy and well-fed babies. At a later period, those who survive infancy, and learn to use their legs, 'run off the fat,' become not only brighter in appearance but more muscular also than during their fat stage."

Breast-fed babies are less liable to become fat than babies fed from the bottle. When babies feed from the breast, they regulate their own intake. When they are fed from the bottle, Mom often determines how much is enough, and what Mom determines is sometimes too much. Unfortunately, overfeeding in infancy can lead to the development of excessive fat cells in the body, and once fat cells make their appearance, they are often there for life. Fat children have a tendency to become fat adults.

Many of these problems can be avoided by deleting cow's milk from the diet. Our dairy herds have been so bred, and they are so fed, that their milk contains a great excess of fat as well as protein. Cow's milk is not even the best milk for the lower animals. Raw goat's milk is superior to that of the cow.

Author Robert S. Mendelsohn, M.D., in *Male Practice: How Doctors Manipulate Women*, recommends the use of mother's milk for infants for another reason. He says: "The bottle-fed baby is much more likely to suffer a nightmare of illnesses that include diarrhea, colic, gastrointestinal and respiratory infections, meningitis, asthma, hives, other allergies, pneumonia, eczema, obesity, arteriosclerosis, dermatitis, growth retardation, hypocalcemic tetany, neonatal hypothyroidism, necrotizing enterocolitis and sudden infant death syndrome. Babies raised on canned formula milk may also be affected by ingesting too much lead."

Babies should always be breast-fed if possible. If Mom does not have sufficient milk, give the baby as much breast milk as there is, and supplement this with cow's or goat's milk. Although human milk is much lower in total protein than cow's milk, it contains much more of the two amino acids cystine and tryptophan, and its protein is much superior to the protein of cow's milk. If the child must be fed wholly on cow's milk, this should be supplemented with fruit juices.

Cow's Milk Is Not the Ideal Food. Milk is adequate for the earliest period of life, but it is inadequate for adults. A diet of fruits, nuts and green vegetables will sustain life, health and growth in adulthood. Whole tribes have lived on such a diet for generations. Author David Reuben, M.D., famous for his *Save Your Life Diet*, says, "More careful analysis of medical records around the world has revealed that when African tribes adopt a Western diet, they gradually develop Western diseases." Milk is not part of the African adult's "deprived" diet.

In the U.S., the mineral and vitamin content of cow's milk vary greatly, perhaps more than those of any other food product. Safe milk depends upon a healthy cow, that has received proper food, sunshine and fresh air, plus clean handling of the milk. Pasteurization does not make unclean milk clean, and to pasteurize milk only further adds to the loss of quality of the vitamins and minerals it contains.

Another factor which renders milk an inadequate food for adults is that it combines poorly with all other foods because of its protein and fat (cream) content. It makes a *fair* combination only with acid fruits. The first thing that occurs when milk enters the stomach is that it coagulates—forms curds. These curds tend to form around particles of other food in the stomach, insulating them against the gastric juices. This prevents their digestion until after the milk curd is digested. Drinking milk is one of the reasons that many adults become overweight.

Health advocate and Hygienist Alec Burton, D.O., D.C. has observed the quick action taken by the body when milk is consumed. Much mucus is secreted, and diseases associated with mucous membranes such as asthma, sinusitis or bronchitis are aggravated. Dr. Burton said in an article, "Milk," in *Dr. Shelton's Hygienic Review*, "Milk is often considered a major source of the vital element calcium: If we don't drink milk, our teeth will fall out and our bones collapse, or some such nonsense. Calcium is abundant in nature. Most of the foods, fruits, vegetables and nuts we recommend are excellent sources of calcium. It would have to be a very poor diet indeed that did not supply half a gram of calcium daily. A good Hygienic diet would provide in excess of one gram."

"Our teeth will fall out" or "our bones will collapse" are not the only false claims made for the virtues of drinking milk. Most of the supposed curative virtues of an exclusive milk diet are also false. Milk contains no excess of vitamins or minerals that will compensate for the use of devitalized foods. Whole milk produces constipation in about 80 percent of those who drink it and diarrhea in perhaps 10 percent. It causes much gas and abdominal discomfort. A diet *strictly* of milk causes increased blood pressure, nausea in many, bowel inaction in a few, catarrh in many, and places a heavy burden on the heart, liver, stomach, intestines, kidneys, lungs and glands. Most patients gain weight rapidly on milk, but such weight is not a gain in healthy flesh and is almost never permanent. Milk has completely wrecked many patients.

If milk is to be taken at all in adulthood, it is best taken alone. Second best is with acid fruits.

RULES FOR TAKING BEVERAGES

1. Do not drink water *with* meals, but rather about half an hour before meals so that the water does not dilute the digestive process.

2. Drink all the water desired *thirty minutes* after a fruit meal, *two* hours after a starch meal, *four* hours after a protein meal.

3. Drink water in response to your body's natural needs. No rigid rules can be set down in regard to how much is too often.

4. Do not drink alcohol, coffee, tea or carbonated beverages.

5. Fruit and/or vegetable juices are best taken one-half hour before a meal and should correctly combine with the meal.

6. Take milk (if at all, goat's or buttermilk) alone or with acid fruits.

::::::::::::::::::::::::::::

PART TWO

THE HYGIENIC
WEIGHT-LOSS PROGRAM

I humbled my soul with fasting.

PSALM 69:10

::

CHAPTER FIVE

THE OPTIONAL START: FOR THE DESPERATE DIETER

AN OPTIONAL WAY to begin this diet consists of a total fast followed by a juice feast. We have included fasting in our dieting program because some people find this method an easier way to switch over to eating natural foods. It is not easy for the habitual user of processed foods, sugar, coffee, salt and so forth, to change to new eating habits. The fast may be useful in helping to clear a previously distorted sense of taste. Another advantage of a fast is that it quells the desire for food.

Also, "Fasting facilitates elimination of toxic wastes and promotes efficient utilization of nutrients," says Hygienist and health advocate Vivian V. Vetrano, B.S., D.C., M.D., in the publication *Healthful Living* (Vol. II, No. 5, 1983). According to Dr. Vetrano, drug use and other unhealthful practices cause cell wall damage, resulting in impaired nutrition. "Fasting enables the body to repair damaged cells, thus improving its nutritive processes."

Some praise the total fast and juice feast as a successful way to lose weight, while others (particularly compulsive overeaters) prefer to cut down on their food intake rather than making such a sudden, drastic change. It's true that when the fast is over, the dieter has not learned new eating habits to help maintain the weight loss. If you "make up for lost time" by overeating after the fast, the detrimental effects of the sudden basic system changes are harder on your body than sustained overweight.

Author Kelly D. Brownell, Ph.D., of the University of Pennsylvania in Philadelphia, who counsels dieters and their spouses, claims continual losing and regaining of weight can be harmful. In her book, *The Partnership Diet Program,* Dr. Brownell says, "Blood pressure and serum cholesterol can increase abnormally during periods of weight gain, and may not return to normal during weight loss."

Overeating after a fast is harmful. If you feel you do not have the discipline to attempt a total fast or a juice feast and you feel fasting is not for you, skip Chapter Five and proceed to Chapter Six.

Start your diet with Week One. Note that this optional fasting week can be referred to and followed at any time. If you choose to start with Week One, and then later on decide to fast, this is certainly permissible. But do understand that nothing is gained by slowly easing into a program of dieting. You will lose weight sooner if the change is made as quickly and abruptly as possible. There is no immediate danger to life as a result of the sudden breaking off of a habit, long practiced, although it may be followed by one or more crises more or less severe, as the organism accommodates itself to the changing conditions of eliminating toxins from the body. Because a habit does not seem to be immediately destructive is no evidence that it is not destructive, or that it is beneficial. Its secondary effects alone can furnish the clue to its influence. A cup of coffee produces an immediate feeling of wellbeing, while no such feeling accompanies a glass of orange juice. But when the secondary effects of these two substances are viewed, no room for doubt is left as to which of these is really beneficial and which is injurious.

THE TOTAL FAST

The first three days of the program call for total fasting on distilled water. When you fast, you voluntarily abstain from all food except pure water, giving rest to the entire body. When digestion and assimilation of food are suspended, the elimination of toxins is increased. Blood pressure decreases and the process of healing is facilitated. Aging and sick cells are renewed and regenerated, providing disease has not reached an irreversible stage. Excess fat and abnormal deposits are consumed as food during the fast, while the cells and tissues of vital organs are preserved. You can expect to lose not less than a pound and a half per day during the first three days of fasting. Some people, particularly men, will lose more than that, although much of this is a loss of fluid weight and not a reduction of actual fat. The more you weigh when you begin the fast, the more weight you can expect to lose during it.

Use distilled water rather than tap water or mineral

water, because distilled water is water in its purest form. Hard waters and mineral waters contain considerable amounts of heavy metals such as copper and lead, and are injurious in proportion to the amount of minerals they contain. That waters high in mineral content do contain substances that are unfriendly to life is obvious from their effect upon the hands that are much washed in such water. Yet the skin of the hands is firmer and more resistant to irritation than the delicate membrane which lines the digestive tract and the lining of the internal surfaces of the arteries and veins. When mineral waters are first taken in, the irritation they set up causes diarrhea. But as their use is continued, thickening and hardening of the lining of the digestive tract occurs as a protective reaction and the diarrhea ceases. A similar hardening and thickening takes place in the arteries and veins. Distilled water causes no such irritation. But it is not "dead" (water is never alive), nor does it leach minerals from the body.

Ideally, drink water that is as close as possible to body temperature, neither extremely hot nor cold. Taking crushed ice during your fast is not ideal.

Drink only when thirsty during your fast. Drinking huge amounts of water will not help you to lose more weight, nor will it help to detoxify your body. At least two or more eight-ounce glasses are recommended daily. Do not take anything other than distilled water during the fast. Your body will call upon its own natural reserves as certain nutrients are needed.

An interesting experiment performed on dogs has demonstrated the fact that animals actually lived longer when fasting on only water than when inferior substances were added to their diet. Over one hundred years ago in Paris, Dr. J. Magendie gave one pen of dogs a diet of white flour and water, fed a second pen of dogs beef tea, and fasted a third pen of dogs, giving them only water. The water-fed dogs, although they lost considerable weight, were alive long after all members of the two other groups had died. The dogs that were given only water were later fed and all recovered. This occurred because the body feeds upon its own balanced food reserves when no other food is eaten, whereas the body has no adequate provision for meeting the exigencies created by prolonged subsistence on a one-sided diet.

While animal experimentation such as Magendie's adds to our knowledge of nutrition, human metabolism differs from that of animals, and experimental tests made on animals are not necessarily valid for human nutrition. Also, experimental diets are almost never the normal diets of animals in nature or the diets of people. We can conclude in general, however, that foods and combinations of food which are inadequate and unsatisfactory in feeding animals are equally inadequate and unsatisfactory in feeding humans. Taking only distilled water during a fast is more beneficial than attempting to add single-article supplements. When these supplementary substances are taken, you are no longer fasting.*

On the first day of your three-day fast you will discover that you have extra time. Take a sunbath or a walk in the fresh air, answer that letter you filed last month, or buy a book on exercise. During this newfound free time, you may also notice that you do not

---

*Taking vitamin and mineral supplements is not recommended during a fast or during the weight-loss program.

feel topnotch. You may experience a few aches, a head-ache, for example, or dizziness. Don't be alarmed. This is a common experience. It is part of the cleansing process. If you have been used to smoking or taking stimulating food and drink, the more you have in-dulged in these things, the more intense discomfort you may feel. If your body has been abused for many years and you suddenly stop harmful eating and living habits, good health does not follow instantaneously. (If this were to happen, it would seem to indicate that disobedience to the laws of Nature is not really harm-ful after all.) So ignore minor discomforts in view of the health rewards ahead.

Rest is the key. The fast is *not* just abstinence from food—physiologic rest. Fasting means resting on three levels: physiological, physical and psychological. So, during your fast, don't take strenuous exercise, go to work, or experience distress, overstimulation or activ-ity that would exhaust the nervous system in any way.

Only in this way can all the energies of the body be concentrated on detoxification of the cells.

Breaking the Fast. Hygienist Ralph C. Cinque, D.C., director of the Hygeia Health Retreat in Yorktown, Texas and supervisor of thousands of fasts, has found that it is not necessary to employ juices to break a two- or three-day fast. Dr. Cinque says a short fast (seven days or less) can be broken by eating small amounts of succulent fruit (melon is a good choice) every three or four hours throughout the day. In the case of longer fasts, however, no solid food is used to break the fast. Instead, slowly sip four to six ounces of freshly squeezed orange juice, watermelon juice, apple juice or carrot/celery juice. Different kinds of juice may be alternated and taken at intervals of every two to four hours throughout the day. For more information regarding longer fasts, see *Fasting Can Save Your Life* by Herbert M. Shelton or *Fasting for the Health of it* by H. M. Shelton and Jean Oswald, found in the bibliography.

THE JUICE FEAST

Since quick weight loss is desired in this optional week, we recommended that you carry out the remainder of the week taking only juice. Many find that taking just juice for a period of time, rather than taking whole foods, leaves them less hungry. If you eat whole fruits, this engages the digestive enzymes to digest the pulp of the whole fruit, therefore stimulating the appetite for more food. Unlike the total fast, which will probably leave you with a complete absence of desire for food, the juice may only somewhat lessen your desire for food. While on your juice feast, you can continue your normal activities, within moderate bounds.

Fruits and vegetables, of course, are not ideal when they are juiced; however, in special cases of obesity, juice is recommended. All fruits and vegetables lose their nutritional value when they are cut, sliced, blended or juiced. Be careful not to peel the fruits and vegetables and then let them stand out on the counter. They will further lose their flavor and undergo oxidation. Drink the juice fresh each time you make it. Do not prepare it ahead of time and store it in the refrigerator.

The following recipes fill approximately a six- or eight-ounce glass. To lose weight, keep your total intake under twenty-four ounces per day. This amount may be divided into two or three juice "meals" during the day. If you are used to taking something before bedtime, then cut down on your mealtime allowance. You may do this with all of the menus on the succeeding pages. Eating many small meals is not encouraged, but do what you must to stay on the program.

JUICE FEAST RECIPES

Cucumber and Tomato Juice
  2 medium tomatoes
  4 ounces cucumber
Blend in blender.

Vegetable Juice
  3 medium carrots
  3 stalks celery
  2 romaine lettuce leaves
Use a juicer.

Tomato and Celery Juice
  2 medium tomatoes
  3 stalks celery
  parsley (optional)
Use a juicer.

Celery and Apple Juice
  2 small apples
  3 stalks celery
Use a juicer.

Fruit Drink
  ½ papaya
  1 peeled orange
  1 medium apple
  1 pineapple slice (1½ inches)
Blend in blender.

Carrot Vegetable Juice
  ½ pepper, red or green
  4 medium-size carrots
  ½ cucumber
Use a juicer.

Orange-Pineapple Juice
  2 peeled oranges
  1 pineapple slice (3 inches)
Blend in blender.

Blended Avocado Salad
  ½ avocado
  1 tomato
  1 red or green pepper
  3 leaves spinach or cabbage
Use a juicer or blender.

Banana Drink
  2 medium-size bananas
  small amount of distilled
    water
Blend in blender.

OPTIONAL WEEK MENUS

THE TOTAL FAST AND THE JUICE FEAST

Morning	Noon	Evening

Day 1
Distilled water --

Day 2
Distilled water --

Day 3
Distilled water --

Day 4 — *Breaking your fast.*

4 ounces orange juice	6 ounces tomato and celery juice	8 ounces carrot vegetable juice. If desired, 6 ounces watermelon juice before bedtime.

Day 5 — *Total juice in one day not to exceed 24 ounces.*

8 ounces fruit drink	8 ounces cucumber and tomato juice	8 ounces vegetable drink

Day 6

6 ounces orange-pineapple juice	6 ounces carrot-vegetable juice	10 ounces blended avocado salad

Day 7

6 ounces watermelon juice	8 ounces vegetable juice	6 ounces goat's milk or buttermilk

If you wish to fast two days instead of three, skip Day Three and move on to Day Four. All juices are interchangeable, depending on the available fresh fruits and vegetables in season. Do not use juice for more than three days.

Thank God for Herbert Shelton for having written his book.
JUDY MAZEL
TV Interview—1982

CHAPTER SIX

WEEK ONE: FRUITS AND VEGETABLES

THE FIRST TWO DAYS of the diet in Week One consist of the mono-meal—consisting of one fruit only— and correctly combined fruit meals. Make an entire meal of fruits. A fruit meal will not cause the troubles that arise from eating fruits with bacon, eggs, toast and denatured foods, nor will it demoralize digestion. Experience the joy of eating such a nourishing good meal and the comfortable feeling that follows. Nothing is more refreshing than eating a delicious apple, a luscious, well-ripened pineapple, a juicy orange or a sweet mango.

Fruits are not only fun to see, to smell and to taste— they are full of sugars and champion flavor-blends of acids, minerals and vitamins. For example:

An apple is a rich source of calcium, phosphorus, sulfur, iron and magnesium. Its phosphoric acid is in the most soluble form, while the iron in the apple is more easily taken into the blood than iron from any other source.

A good California avocado contains amounts of amino acids comparable to those in milk. It offers liberal supplies of vitamins, minerals and fats in their natural state. The natural fat in avocado has not been found to raise uric acid or cholesterol levels above normal.

A fully ripened banana (one that is flecked with little brown spots) is about equal in protein value to grains and potatoes. It is almost predigested and it is rich in vitamins A, B, D, and high in potassium. There is little doubt that an adult could live for some time on bananas alone without any appreciable decrease in strength or health.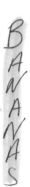

The date is richer in protein than most fruits (varying in this element from 1.3 percent to over 2 percent).

The mineral content of figs closely resembles that of mother's milk.

Oranges are rich in lime and other alkaline salts. Their use combats acidosis and prolongs youth. These, with grapefruit, are the best agents to eat if you are ill. Be sure they are tree-ripened; try to buy organically grown.

The tomato ranks next to the orange in its beneficial effects. It is the equal of oranges both in vitamins (they both contain much vitamin A and C), and in alkaline elements.

The papaya has a high vitamin content—per 100 grams it contains 2,500 units of vitamin A, 33 units of vitamin B and 70 units of vitamin C.

Not only are fruits nutritious foods but they are superior to starch as a source of carbohydrates. Sweet fruits serve the same heat and energy purposes in the body that starch does, and need almost no digestion. Digesting starch foods consumes much more energy than digesting sweet fruits, which give the greatest amount of nourishment for the least amount of digestive strain. Starch must be converted into sugar before the body can use it. Fruit sugars have already been converted from starch to sugar while ripening under the sun. The sun and the life force of the tree do this work for you. You will lose weight more quickly and save your energy when you eat fruit instead of eating cereals, potatoes, bread and other starchy foods.

Although fruits are the choicest of all foods, they are not complete foods. *No one should attempt to live exclusively upon fruits.* They are usually lacking in complex albumin. Most of them are low in calcium and many of them are deficient in vitamin A. Few of them are rich in protein—the avocado and olive being the chief exceptions. Therefore, fruits should not be eaten exclusively for a period longer than one month. But for special purposes such as dieting, their use makes an ideal beginning to a weight-loss program.

Be sure to wash your fruits carefully in cool water before eating them. Apples, in particular, are often excessively sprayed. They are best peeled before eating, unless organically grown. Savor each bite! Take your time in eating fruits. Be very leery about eating unripe fruits. They contain starch and other carbohydrate substances that are unwholesome. On the other hand, if the fruits are overripe, the sugar is changed into carbon dioxide, alcohol and acetic acid, and loses its wholesomeness. Experience will teach you to know when each fruit is just right for eating.

HOW TO COMBINE FRUITS

Fruits fall into three classifications, acid, sub-acid and sweet, and combine best with other fruits in their own classification. Sub-acid and acid fruits combine fairly well, but acid and sweet fruits combine poorly. Miscombining fruits will cause indigestion, gas and other discomforts.

FRUIT CLASSIFICATION

Acid Fruits

acerola	loganberry	sour peach
currant	orange	sour plum
grapefruit	pineapple	strawberry
kumquat	pomegranate	tamarind
lemon	sour apple	tangerine
lime	sour grape	tomato

Sub-acid Fruits

apple	fresh fig	nectarine
apricot	grape	papaya
blackberry	huckleberry	pawpaw
cherimoya	kiwi	peach
cherry (ripe and	mango	pear
sweet)	mangosteen	raspberry
elderberry	mulberry	sweet plum

Sweet Fruits

banana	muscat grape	Thompson grape
carob	persimmon	
cherimoya	prune	all dried fruits
date	raisin	such as pears,
fig	sapodilla	apricots, etc.

We put melons in a special classification because they undergo little or no digestion in the mouth and stomach. Melons pass quickly into the intestine where they undergo the little digestion they require. To eat them with other foods that require more digestion time means that the melon will remain in the stomach until the completion of the digestion of the other foods. Bacterial decomposition follows. If your digestion is good, you may combine melons with acid or sub-acid fruits; however, do not combine melons with sweet fruits.

Melons

banana melon	Crenshaw melon	nutmeg melon
cantaloupe	honeydew	Persian melon
casaba	muskmelon	pie melon
Christmas melon		watermelon

Another fruit which requires special handling is the avocado. The avocado contains equal protein to that of milk and is rich in fat. Combining avocados with acid and sub-acid is acceptable; the fat contained in the avocado inhibits the secretion of gastric juice as much and as long as do acids. However, when the avocado is eaten with sweet fruits, the high sugar content of the fruit interferes with the digestion of proteins contained in the avocado. Fermentation follows this combination.

To insure good digestion, observe certain rules when eating fruits:

1. Make an entire meal of fruits.
2. All fruits combine best when they are combined with other fruits in the same classification.
3. Melons are best eaten alone.
4. Do not combine acid fruits—or avocados—with sweet fruits.
5. Do not eat more than the required amounts of fruit listed in our proposed menus. Eating excessive amounts of fruit will result in loose stools.

How Many Meals per Day? When dieting, we recommend that you eat two meals per day. In fact, after you are down to your desired weight, you may want to continue eating two meals each day. We feel two meals daily are better than three unless the three meals are very small. Eating three meals with a midafternoon snack and a late evening snack keeps a steady stream of food pouring into the intestine. If the meals are small, the intestine may not have to work harder but it certainly does not work less. The circulatory system must keep this food moving. The liver must store certain surpluses, while the kidneys and bowels are at work. All meals, whether light or heavy, whether taken morning, noon or night, or between these times, cause blood and nerve energy to be shuttled to the digestive organs and away from the brain and muscles. Instead of immediately yielding up energy, eating uses stored energy in the work of digesting food. With small, frequent meals, the glands of the mouth and stomach receive less rest. "Little and often" is not in our plan;

it does not provide adequate rest for the digestive apparatus.

There is an added health benefit to eating two meals each day. A great number of sick individuals and invalids have regained their health on two meals per day. The rest provides the condition for impaired organs and functions to heal and become more efficient. Life can be prolonged under this plan. In the 1600s, one Luigi Cornaro lived to be 102, eating two meals a day. And these meals were small. He ate no more than fourteen ounces of food each day.

The Mono-Meal. The mono-fruit meal, eating only one fruit at a meal, brings ultimate simplicity to eating. Try the mono-meal and you will discover you will lose weight. When one food is eaten at a meal there is always greater efficiency of digestion. Although eating occasional mono-meals is good for digestion and is a good way to lose weight, this does not mean that we advocate following a mono-diet for a period longer than one month. Diets such as the "grape diet" bombard the body with too much sugar. Eating mono-meals for longer than thirty days will prove inadequate to meet the body's total requirements. The deficiencies of one foodstuff should be supplemented by an abundance of the deficient factors in another food. But *occasional* mono-meals are ideal when dieting.

There is another benefit to eating only one food at a meal. Some people find their hunger is satisfied sooner than if they eat a variety of foods. If you eat only one type of fruit, you eat just so much and are satisfied, because you gratify the needs of the cells (*hunger*) rather than *appetite*. If you eat two fruits, you tend to eat as much of each as you would of a single fruit. For example, if you eat all you want of pineapple, you might go back for a few oranges or kiwi and start eating all over again. Variety is the spice of gluttony. This common experience does not prove that you need a variety of foods to supply your body's demands at the time; it does prove that a variety of foods leads to overeating.

Use the mono-meal to try this experiment in distinguishing between *hunger* and *appetite*, two terms with completely different meanings. Use only one food—any food will do. In the following example, we use a large bunch of bananas.

It is time for your meal—your stomach is rumbling so you hurriedly peel the banana. Suddenly you remember that you are supposed to eat slowly, chew thoroughly and have reverence for your food. Therefore, you quiet yourself, slow down, and enjoy the banana. The second one tastes just as good. The third one is not quite as exciting, but you know it is all you are going to eat so you slow down even more. You eat the fourth banana very reluctantly and decide you have had enough. Twenty minutes later you proclaim that you are hungry. "Well, I'll have another banana," exclaims an inner voice; however, in the next sentence the voice says, "But I don't want a banana."

This is where appetite takes over. The biological need is filled (you are *not* hungry!) but the psychological need for *stimulation* takes over (you have an appetite).

Understanding the difference between appetite and hunger will help you to analyze what it is you *really* want. It's not food! Is the desire caused by boredom? A need for love? Review the list of reasons why you overeat on page 8. Not until you understand and overcome that elusive need will you gain a sense of freedom from the habit of stimulating yourself with food.

What About Breakfast? How much energy do you derive from starting the day with breakfast? None! Food requires up to four hours (depending on what type of food and combinations are eaten) to complete stomach digestion. When the food passes from the stomach to the intestine, several more hours are needed for digestion to be completed. You do not receive energy from food while it is still in the stomach and intestine being digested. When the food finally reaches the cells by way of the blood, then the body builds energy.

The food energy with which you start the day is derived from the food eaten the day before, or the week before, or even the month before. Food stores in the body are always available for instant use, if you miss one or several meals. The food eaten the preceding evening is not all used up by the little energy expended while sleeping. The night's rest is the preparation for the next day's activity.

A large breakfast or lunch very often gives a person a sluggish, tired feeling. This definitely prevents many people from carrying on their work efficiently and actively in the afternoon.

Try the no-breakfast plan and see how you feel. This may be contrary to the rules that go with other weight-loss programs. We are aware that many advocate that you not skip meals while you are trying to lose weight because there is a tendency to overeat on the next meal. On the contrary, you might be surprised to discover that you may not desire more food at noontime. If our two-meal-a-day plan does not work out for you and you must have breakfast, divide the noon meal into two smaller meals—one for breakfast and one for lunch.

WEEK ONE, DAY THREE: ADDING THE VEGETABLES

Until the discovery of vitamins no one, except the students of natural feeding practices, knew why the gentle old cow would occasionally smash fences to get into the growing alfalfa or on the other side where the grass was green. Give the cow access to both green vegetation and grains, and the cow will eat most heavily of the greens.

Men, women and children require daily supplies of green vegetation as much as certain animals do. These needs are not met by eating a few leaves of lettuce, a slice of tomato, a radish or a pickled olive. Such a salad is not worthy of the name and would only meet the salad needs of a canary. You need to eat a tubful of it. A big salad can be the most enjoyable and valuable food on a diet program, whether to lose weight or maintain desired weight.

But not all people are interested in including raw vegetables in their diet. Some complain that they cannot take so much of what they call "roughage" or "fiber foods," perhaps better termed "bulk." (An explanation of the facts is found in *Food Combining Made Easy* by Dr. Shelton, listed in the bibliography.) The complaint that vegetables contain too much roughage or fiber is not based on fact. The harm is done by a diet heavy in meats and cereals. Conventional eaters who eat flesh, eggs and cereals actually have more of an urgent need for one or two green leafy vegetable salads daily than the person who lives largely on raw fruits and vegetables. There are no substitutes for green leafy salads. Fruits cannot take their place.

Author Arnold Fox, M.D. advises eating vegetables to help prevent cancer. He says that cancer is related to what people do and do not eat. The exact mechanism of diet's relationship to cancer is still shrouded in mystery, but it is known that there are at least two steps involved—initiation and activation.

A normal cell is initiated when a carcinogen alters the cell's DNA (the genetic master plan). Certain foods, chemicals, ultraviolet light, radiation, pickled foods and nitrates, when added to food, are initiators. The initiated cell may remain dormant for minutes, days, years or decades. It will not cause problems unless it is activated. Substances known as activators can wake up the sleeping initiated cell, turning it into a dangerous cell. These cells use the nutrients in the body to grow until they crowd, invade and take over.

The activating substances are fats (animal fats) and vegetable oils.

The key to reducing the risks of cancer, claims Dr. Fox, is to adopt a low-fat, high-complex carbohydrate diet, stop smoking, keep your weight at its optimal level, stop or reduce coffee consumption, stop or reduce intake of additives, and eat crucifers and foods rich in beta-carotene.

Members of the crucifer family include common vegetables such as cabbage, brussels sprouts, cauliflower, kale, collards, turnips and kohlrabi. Beta-carotenes are

::::::::::::::::::::::::::

a group of yellow-colored compounds found in carrots, sweet potatoes, dark green vegetables, orange vegetables and oranges. Dr. Fox calls these anti-cancer foods.

Fresh vegetables, preferably raw, help reduce the risk of cancer. Here are a few more facts you should know about the nutritional value of green and other vegetables:

Green leafy vegetables (which usually contain more abundant alkaline minerals than fruits) are richly supplied with sodium, calcium, organic salts and vitamins A and C. They are the best sources of chlorophyll and are also sources of small quantities of the highest-grade protein and trace minerals, all in the proper proportions and balance for the body to use in making "replacement parts" (the cells).

Greener leaves

The outer, greener leaves and stalks of lettuce, celery and cabbage contain more vitamins and minerals than the white inner leaves and stalks.

Cucumbers are rich in iron, potash, magnesium, calcium and vitamin C. They are best eaten whole, seeds, skin (if unwaxed) and all. Their skins are rich in minerals valuable to the body.

Green Pepper

A green pepper contains seven times more vitamin C than an orange.

Vegetables that grow above ground in the sun tend to contain more vitamins and minerals than vegetables that grow under ground.

Beet tops, radish tops and turnip tops are more important foods than beets, radishes and turnips.

A two-pound head of cabbage contains more organic salts of iodine than the thyroid gland can use in a week.

Spinach, beet tops, turnip tops, kale, mustard, dandelion and leeks all have similar, excellent food value (spinach is not superior, as commonly assumed).

Iceberg lettuce is harder to digest and has less food value than leaf lettuce.

If green leafy lettuce is shredded, it may lose as much as 80 percent of its vitamin C in one minute.

To derive the maximum nutritional value from green vegetables, they are best home-grown without using pesticides. But if you must purchase them at a market, choose only the fresh, crisp vegetables. Wilted, shrunken vegetables have lost both palatability and nutritional value.

The green outer leaves of plants that are exposed to the sunlight make the finest salads. Lettuce, celery, cucumbers, tomatoes, green and red peppers (the non-pungent varieties) and cabbage make excellent salad vegetables. Raw turnip greens, young radish leaves and spinach also make tasty and valuable additions to salads. Such foods as raw onions (steamed onions are less objectionable), garlic, watercress and radishes are not recommended for salads.

When you make salads, don't soak the vegetables in water. Rather, rinse them thoroughly, taking care not to bruise them. Soaking vegetables in water leaches minerals and vitamins from them and reduces their food value. The processes of shredding, dicing, cutting and slicing vegetables and fruits permits the air to reach them, and this also results in loss and destruction of vitamins. The finer a vegetable is chopped or the longer it is soaked in water, the greater the vitamin loss.

Chopping vegetables sometimes tempts you to put the whole garden into a salad. Keep the salad simple. The object in making a salad is not to see how many ingredients can be mixed together. Three or four vegetables are sufficient.

The following recipes are not intended to exhaust the list of delightful salads that you might make. They are intended, rather, to serve as guides to improvising.

¼ romaine lettuce
1 bunch of parsley
1 sweet pepper
1 whole tomato

½ head lettuce
1 whole tomato
3 stalks celery

¼ pound leaf lettuce
1 whole cucumber
2 stalks fennel
    from the fennel root

¼ head cabbage
green beans
bean sprouts

¼ head cabbage
fresh peas
1 stalk French endive

¼ pound radish leaves
1 large tomato
3 stalks celery
lemon juice

¼ pound fresh spinach
3 stalks green celery
Chinese cabbage
1 red pepper

¼ pound chard
raw broccoli
2 whole carrots

1 head endive (chicory)
asparagus spears
1 green pepper

¼ pound turnip leaves
fresh young corn
1 whole cucumber

¼ pound dandelion leaves
2 carrots
2 stalks celery
1 stalk endive

mixed salad of Bibb lettuce
   and kale
½ avocado
1 tomato
2 carrots

Eating vegetable salads doesn't have to become boring. Many combinations are possible. Invent your own from any of the following raw vegetables:

alfalfa sprouts	chives	okra
anise	collards	parsley
asparagus	corn (young)	peas
bamboo shoots	dandelion	red peppers
basil	eggplant	redtip lettuce
Bibb lettuce	endive	romaine lettuce
beets	escarole	scallions
beet tops (greens)	fennel	sorrel
broccoli	green beans	spinach
brussels sprouts	green pepper	summer squash
cabbage	kale	Swiss chard
cardoon	kohlrabi	tomatoes
carrots	lettuce	turnip
cauliflower	mullein	watercress
celery	mung bean sprouts	zucchini
chicory	mustard greens	

Although it is preferable to eat your salad without dressings so as not to mask the delicate flavors, a simple dressing of lemon juice or avocado (blended with water) may be added. The salad dressings listed below are suitable when the salad is eaten alone or when it is followed by steamed green vegetables. The recipes—each for two dieters—are in reduced quantities for a weight-loss program. If you wish to maintain your weight, you may increase the amounts.

::::::::::::::::::::::::::

Avocado-Tomato Dressing

   1 medium avocado, peeled
   2 cherry tomatoes
   2 tablespoons celery juice
Blend in blender.

Tomato Dressing

   2 medium-size tomatoes
   1 green or red pepper
   small avocado
Blend in blender.

Avocado-Pepper Dressing

   1 medium avocado, peeled
   2 tablespoons celery juice
   1 green or red pepper
Blend in blender.

The third day of the diet is simple. One meal consists of fruits and the other, a large raw salad. The salad can be followed by one or two steamed vegetables. Keep the amount of steamed vegetables under two cups. You don't need to eat them every day. When you have reached your desired weight, you may eat as much as you like of steamed vegetables. Do *not* boil them; steam them instead, as little as possible to retain their fiber. Fiber in foods adds extra volume to the contents of the gastrointestinal tract. In return you will feel satisfied with less food; thorough chewing also satisfies hunger pangs.

STEAMING CHART

Vegetable and Quantity (1 pound, *except as noted*)	*Approx. Minutes*	*Classification*
beans, string	12–15	green
broccoli	10	green
brussels sprouts	10	non-starchy
cabbage (green or red) 1 head	10–15	non-starchy
celery	10	green

Vegetable and Quantity (1 pound, except as noted)	Approx. Minutes	Classification
chard	5	non-starchy
collards	5	non-starchy
eggplant, sliced 1 large	5–10	non-starchy
fennel	5–8	non-starchy
kale	5–8	non-starchy
kohlrabi	10–15	non-starchy
okra	5	green
parsnips, sliced	10	non-starchy
peas, green shelled	5	legume
peas, pods (snow)	5	legume
peppers, green, 4 large	5–8	green
spinach	5	green
squash (zucchini)	15–20	non-starchy
tomato	5–8	acid

RULES FOR EATING VEGETABLES

1. Make your salads of fresh, raw vegetables.
2. To avoid a loss of vitamins and minerals, don't soak vegetables in water.
3. Use vegetables whole or cut into large pieces.
4. Keep your salads simple. Three or four ingredients are sufficient.
5. You may put lemon on a salad when it is eaten alone or is followed by two steamed, non-starchy or green vegetables. (Dressings need not always be included in the salad.)

As a variation, a tasty meal may be made of a fruit salad, but only a few vegetables go well with fruits. The vegetables that can be combined with anything—fruits, protein or starch—we call neutral vegetables.

The list of neutral vegetables is followed by sample recipes for fruit salads.

NEUTRAL VEGETABLES

Bibb lettuce	endive	redtip lettuce
celery	green pepper	romaine lettuce
chicory	kale	Swiss chard
cucumber	lettuce	
dandelion	parsley	

FRUIT SALADS

½ grapefruit	1 apple
1 orange	2 ounces grapes
1 slice pineapple	1 slice pineapple
celery	celery
lettuce	romaine lettuce

2 ounces cherries	3 apricots
1 nectarine	2 ounces grapes
1 plum	1 peach
celery	celery
lettuce	lettuce
½ avocado	

Do not follow a fruit salad with steamed vegetables.

MENUS FOR WEEK ONE

Spring and Summer
Fruits and Vegetables

	Noon	*Evening*
MONDAY (mono-meals)		
	watermelon (as much as desired)	3 peaches or more

	Noon	*Evening*
TUESDAY		
	Ripe pineapple (as much as desired but not to exceed 1 whole pineapple)	2 pears 4 ounces Bing cherries
WEDNESDAY		
	5 ounces grapes ¼ avocado	large vegetable salad
THURSDAY		
	fruit salad	large vegetable salad dressing
FRIDAY		
	3 or more apples	broccoli vegetable salad
SATURDAY		
	up to six tomatoes	vegetable salad brussels sprouts zucchini
SUNDAY		
	grapes (not to exceed ¾ pounds)	vegetable salad okra green beans

Naturally, the less food you eat, the faster you will lose weight. Hypoglycemics should avoid fruit juices and meals consisting of all fruits, as well as avoiding all dried fruits. An avocado will assist in stabilizing the blood sugar level when eaten with fruits.

The menus for week one can be followed for up to one month, if you desire to do so, but do not exceed four weeks.

::::::::::::::::::::::::::::

MENUS FOR WEEK ONE

Fall and Winter
Fruits and Vegetables

	Noon	*Evening*
MONDAY (mono-meals)	honeydew melon (as much as desired)	3 apples or more
TUESDAY (mono-meals)	2 papayas	up to six medium-size tomatoes with small salad
WEDNESDAY	vegetable salad steamed kale	1 medium-size banana 2 ounces unsulfured raisins romaine lettuce steamed parsnips
THURSDAY	1 orange ½ papaya ½ avocado	vegetable salad
FRIDAY	vegetable salad steamed Jerusalem artichoke*	1 mango 1 kiwi fruit ½ avocado
SATURDAY	vegetable salad broccoli	½ papaya 1 pear

*The Hygienic diet consists predominantly of uncooked foods. You will discover that the more raw foods you eat, the faster you will lose weight.

	Noon	*Evening*
SUNDAY	fruit salad	vegetable salad turnip greens zucchini

Note: You will lose the same amount of weight whether you eat a mono-meal or a meal with two fruits or vegetables in the same classification. It is the amount that makes the difference. "Keep the amount of sweet fruits lower than that of the acid and sub-acid fruits because of their higher sugar content," said Hygienic Practitioner David J. Scott, D.O., director of Scott's Natural Health Institute in Cleveland Ohio.

On learning that a patient rejects meat, a doctor may get nervous enough to give what I call the "voodoo curse" of the religion of Modern Medicine, i.e., threatening vitamin B12 deficiency with all its attendant symptoms.

ROBERT S. MENDELSOHN M.D.
The People's Doctor

:::

CHAPTER SEVEN

WEEK TWO:
THE NEW WAY TO EAT PROTEIN

WHEN YOU ARE BUILDING a house, large quantities of building materials are required. Once the house is completed, small quantities of material can keep it in a state of repair. In the same manner, your body requires the greatest amount of building material (protein) while it is growing; once you reach maturity, you need only small quantities of building material for maintenance. It is inconceivable that a great deal of protein is required by an old man or woman who is not growing and whose processes of metabolism have slowed down.

After the age of twenty-five your ability to digest protein diminishes. When growth is completed, Nature provides for the digestion of less protein. The human organism requires a low-protein diet at all ages

:::::::::::::::::::::::::::::::::::

of life, but less protein after maturity. The physical worker requires possibly a little more protein than the sedentary worker. Women require a little more protein during pregnancy and lactation. An additional amount is needed during puberty and adolescence. Men require a small increase during the active reproductive period. Both sexes require more protein after a fast or a wasting illness. If you undergo a course of physical training designed to put on a lot of muscle, more protein is required, but certainly not enormous quantities.

PROTEIN SOURCES

avocado (low protein)
cereals (use sparingly)
cheese (unprocessed and unsalted, preferably soft)
dried beans (protein-starch combo)
dried peas (protein-starch combo)
egg yolk
lentils
meat
milk (low protein)
nuts
olives
peanuts (protein-starch combo)
soybeans

The body stores little protein. Since the excess passes out through the kidneys, a high-protein diet overworks them. There is a definite limit to the amount of protein that can be digested each day. When more protein is eaten than is needed, some is excreted unused, but much of the undigested protein tends to putrefy in the digestive tract and in the colon, resulting in foul stools and toxicity. Excess protein accelerates all the functions of life, and hence tends to exhaust the organism. This is notably true of the sexual function: animals breed more often if overfed on protein and hens lay more eggs on a high-protein diet. (Such a diet does not produce superior offspring.)

The body continues to function in spite of a high-protein diet because of its elaborate system of getting rid of the surplus and toxins. People often assume that the digestive organs are able to reject any injurious substance. Unfortunately, the capacity to do this is limited, and injurious effects sooner or later become evident. Many diseases and deaths are due to an overstrain that causes breakdown of the organs and functions of elimination. Or, more correctly, when the processes of elimination are impaired and the poisons permitted to accumulate, the person sickens and dies from the accumulation of a toxic overload. Overabundance of protein is a curse rather than a boon to the body. You reduce energy by eating too much protein and poison yourself at the same time.

One of the longest experiments employing a low-protein diet was conducted by Mikel Hindhede, M.D., a Food Administrator in Denmark. His experiment covered a period of three years during World War I. Hindhede found in his studies that the less protein in a nation's diet, the less the population suffered from disease. He concluded that the average adult human may require twenty grams of protein daily, but that the requirement may be even less than this. A more recent experiment is reported in *The Vegetarian Handbook* by Rodger Doyle. The test was made in the early 1970s by a group of researchers headed by Dr. B. J. Meyer from the University of Pretoria in South Africa.

Twenty-seven adults were given about two ounces of peanuts, cashews or walnuts and one-half to three-quarters of a pound of avocados each day. The diet also included carrots, tomatoes and fresh or dried fruit. This diet provided adequate nutrients. Dr. Meyer suggests that the diet may have health advantages. Those participants who had previously been overweight slimmed down to their ideal weight during the test.

The participants had lower blood pressure and reductions in serum cholesterol and triglyceride levels (possible signs of lower atherosclerosis risk) after the experiment.

Dr. Meyer and his colleagues conducted an experiment to see if it is possible for trained athletes to run as well on a fruitarian diet as on a conventional meat diet. Nine student runners (between the ages of seventeen and twenty-four) were on a conventional meat diet for a year. During that time they exercised every day for an hour. A high-protein diet was instituted for several weeks, followed by a high-carbohydrate diet for a few days. This was done immediately prior to competition. In the competition they ran an eight-kilometer course. Immediately afterward, the student runners went on a fruitarian diet for two weeks (two-thirds of their calories were carbohydrates). After this they ran the same course and *all* nine runners improved in performance.

These examples are a reminder that the overuse of protein food in the diet is detrimental to health. The cells of most of the body pass through their regular life cycle and are replaced by new ones. Whether they are replaced by normal cells or imperfect cells depends upon what kinds of materials form the new cells, and the amount of cellular waste present. Most cells of the body are constantly created anew, but if blood and lymph chemistry are not normal, the process of renewal is imperfect. The amount and type of food you eat helps to determine health and longevity; make no mistake about that.

NATURE NEVER PRODUCED A SANDWICH

No animal in a state of nature eats such a great variety of foods as humans. Animals do little combining. The meat-eating animal consumes no carbohydrates or acids with his proteins. The lion in the jungle combines his foods very little. The chipmunk, eating nuts, generally eats his fill of nuts without taking other food with them. Birds often eat insects at one time of day, seeds at another.

Biblical study tells us that humans, like the lower animals, may have instinctively avoided wrong food combinations. For example, Moses said to the people of Israel: "Jehovah shall give you in the evening, flesh to eat, and in the morning, bread to the full." This ancient eating practice has been revived today on physiological grounds—eating protein and starch foods at separate meals because it promotes better digestion. The processes of digestion of these types of foods are different; they do not take place with any degree of efficiency in the same digestive cavity at the same time. So foods should be combined properly to assure more efficient digestion.* Better digestion, of course, means better health.

The process of digestion varies according to the type of foods eaten. Note a remarkable fact concerning the work of the digestive glands: the digestive tract can vary its fluids and enzymes to suit the character of the food being digested. The variations in the enzymatic and other constituents of the digestive secretions in the presence of different foods is an effort by the body to

*Information on food allergies from improper food combining is found in *Food Combining Made Easy,* listed in the bibliography.

99

make the digestive juices conform to their requirements of digestion. These variations include changes in the alkalinity and acidity (pH) of the secretions, in the concentration of the enzymes, and in the timing of the secretions to fit them to the different foods.

This adaptation of the juices and their enzyme content to the character of the food eaten is possible, however, with only one food at a time. When several foods are eaten together, conflict with the digestive processes should be a primary concern. If the foods eaten are radically different, they are harder to digest and may not be digested at all. A ham sandwich, hot dog, spaghetti with meatballs, pizza, meat and potatoes, etc., all protein-starch combinations, cannot be handled with efficiency. They are not natural combinations. Nature never produced a bologna sandwich or a hamburger. The digestive juices cannot easily be adapted simultaneously to the needs of two foods of such opposite character as bread and flesh.

Bread, even if eaten alone, is not the ideal food. It is often made of denatured cereals mixed with salt, soda, yeast and lard and subjected to a high degree of cooking temperature. If eaten at two meals a day and mixed indiscriminately with all classes of foods, bread can become one of the chief sources of overweight and sickness.

To avoid eating bread or other starches with a protein is not the only rule for food combining. Hygienists do not recommend eating two different kinds of concentrated proteins at the same meal because each needs different modifications of digestive secretions and different timing of those secretions in order to be efficiently digested. The strongest juice is poured out upon milk in the last hour of digestion, upon flesh in the first hour. Eggs receive the strongest secretion at a different time from either flesh or milk. It is logical, therefore, that these things should not be eaten together.

This does not mean that two different kinds of flesh, for instance chicken and turkey, may not be eaten together or that two different kinds of nuts may not be eaten at the same time; but it certainly means that you should not combine flesh (such as bacon or ham) and eggs. Don't eat eggs and milk, eggs and cheese, cheese and nuts or a submarine sandwich. One protein food at a meal assures greater efficiency in digestion.

Eating commercial sugars, syrups, sweet fruits and honey with proteins also make it difficult for the digestive system. Sweets have an inhibiting effect on the secretion of gastric juice. Fat eaten with a protein produces an even greater inhibiting effect. This means that eating salad oils or avocados at the same meal with protein foods is not recommended.

If you must eat fat with protein, however, you can somewhat offset its inhibiting effect upon digestion by consuming raw green vegetables with the protein. Non-starchy vegetables combine best with meat protein (if you are not a vegetarian). For vegetarians receiving protein from nuts or seeds, these can be eaten with non-starchy vegetables or acid fruits.

RULES FOR PROTEIN COMBINING

1. Eat protein and starch foods at separate meals.
2. Eat only one concentrated protein food at a meal.
3. Do not combine commercial sugars, syrups, sweet fruits or honey with a protein.

4. Eat proteins and fats at separate meals. (Don't put avocado in your salad when you are also eating protein.)

FATS AND FAT

Fat in your food or taken with your food gives you a satisfied, full feeling. You feel less hungry for a longer period of time than if you ate a meal with no fat at all.

But Mcleod's *Physiology in Modern Medicine* says: "Fat has been shown to exert a distinct inhibiting influence on the secretion of gastric juice . . . the presence of oil in the stomach delays the secretion of juice poured out on a subsequent meal of otherwise readily digestible food." This is an important physiological truth few people know about.

Fat in food lessens the amount of chemical secretion poured out, lessens the activity of the gastric glands, lowers the amount of pepsin and hydrochloric acid in the gastric juice and may lower gastric tone by as much as fifty percent. This inhibiting effect may last two or more hours.

While losing weight, go easy on your daily intake of fat or you will be disappointed when you calculate your weight loss. Don't indulge in more than a dab of unsalted butter or eat more than one-half an avocado per day. The less fat you eat the more weight you will lose.

FAT SOURCES

avocados
butter (choose raw and unsalted)
corn oil (not recommended)
cream
fat meats (not recommended)
lard (not recommended)

most nuts
nut or olive oil
  (not recommended)
sesame, soy or sunflower
  oil (not recommended)

RULES FOR COMBINING FATS

Because fat has an inhibiting effect upon the secretion of gastric juice, follow these two rules:

1. Do not eat fats and proteins at the same meal.
2. Do not combine commercial sugars, syrups or sweet fruits with fats.

MENUS FOR WEEK TWO

Spring and Summer
THE NEW WAY TO EAT PROTEIN

	Noon	*Evening*
MONDAY		
	2 pomegranates or other fruit in season	vegetable salad 1 ounce pecans 1 ounce cashews (not roasted, toasted or salted)
TUESDAY		
	1 pear 1 plum	vegetable salad steamed peas steamed kale

	Noon	*Evening*
WEDNESDAY	fruit salad	vegetable salad 2 ounces filberts
THURSDAY	1 peach 1 nectarine	vegetable salad
FRIDAY	fruit salad 2 ounces walnuts or/ 2 ounces unprocessed raw milk cheese	vegetable salad string beans

SATURDAY	½ pint blueberries	vegetable salad
		raw young tender
		  corn (corn is a
		  protein when
		  young)

SUNDAY	1 very ripe pineapple (as much as desired)	vegetable salad 1 apple

Note: Hypoglycemics, don't forget to add ¼ avocado to the all-fruit meals. Adjust the menu to fit your needs in maintaining stable glucose levels.

MENUS FOR WEEK TWO

Fall and Winter

	Noon	*Evening*
MONDAY	1 fully ripened kiwi fruit 3 ounces grapes	vegetable salad 2 ounces almonds

	Noon	*Evening*
TUESDAY	2 tomatoes with a few leaves of romaine lettuce 2 ounces ricotta cheese	vegetable salad zucchini mustard greens
WEDNESDAY	1 apple ½ avocado	vegetable salad
THURSDAY	1 persimmon (not for the hypoglycemic) 2 figs with a few leaves of Bibb lettuce	vegetable salad steamed peas beet greens
FRIDAY	fruit salad	vegetable salad 2 ounces sunflower seeds (if seeds are well tolerated)
SATURDAY	1 medium-size banana (not for the hypoglycemic) 2 dates with a few leaves of redtip lettuce	vegetable salad soy sprouts red cabbage
SUNDAY	1 grapefruit 2 ounces pecans	vegetable salad steamed eggplant

Note that these menus have been created primarily for those who have had some exposure to the concepts of vegetarianism. Following them will help you to come to a more scientific understanding of your body's bio-chemical needs.

Some people who have not been exposed to this knowledge may still be flesh-eaters and may be in a period of transition. Use good judgment in substituting occasional fish or chicken for your protein meals. You may use three ounces of fish or chicken to replace the **av**ocados or nuts at any meal. Be sure to purchase fish from the deep sea, which is less polluted, and meat from organic farms to avoid the poisonous chemicals and drugs so often fed to animals.

If people would only eat right there would be no need for operations.
JOHN H. TILDEN, M.D. (1851–1940)
Pioneer Hygienist

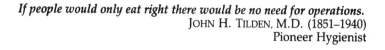

CHAPTER EIGHT

WEEK THREE: ADDING STARCH TO THE DIET

THE LAST WEEK of the weight-loss program includes the addition of starches. Since starch is a carbohydrate food, in order to add it to the program and still lose weight, you just eat less fruit or a little less protein on the days you prepare starch meals.

As mentioned earlier, starch carbohydrates do not digest as easily as fruit carbohydrates. Starch foods, particularly grains, should be used sparingly and with caution, if they are used at all. Cereals take longer to digest than other starch foods. Cereal or grain starches require from eight to twelve times as long to digest as does potato starch. About two hours are required to digest the starch of wheat, corn and rice and eighty minutes to digest the starch of oats, whereas the same amount of potato starch digests in ten minutes.

Mildly starchy vegetables, however, present no problem to the dieter. Even potatoes and yams are included. Potatoes are not fattening if you eat them with green vegetables and limit or omit the butter.

Examples of starch foods are listed below.

STARCH CLASSIFICATION

Mildly Starchy

beets	corn	salsify
carrots	Jerusalem artichokes	turnips
cauliflower	rutabaga	

Starchy

banana squash	dry beans (protein-	peanuts (protein-
caladium root	starch combo)	starch combo)
cauliflower	(except soy beans)	potatoes (all
cereals (use	dry peas (protein-	kinds)
sparingly)	starch combo)	pumpkin
chestnuts	Hubbard squash	salsify

STEAMING CHART

Vegetable and quantity (1 pound, except as noted)	Approx. time	Classification
artichoke (Jerusalem) 3 pounds	30–40 min.	mildly starchy
beets	30–40 min.	mildly starchy
carrots, sliced	10–15 min.	mildly starchy
cauliflower	10 min.	mildly starchy
corn 4 ears	10 min.	mildly starchy
potatoes, white 4 whole	30–40 min.	starchy
potatoes, sweet 4 whole	30–40 min.	starchy
rutabaga	10–15 min.	mildly starchy
salsify	10–15 min.	mildly starchy
squash (butternut) 2 pounds	25–30 min.	starchy
turnips	15–20 min.	mildly starchy

CORRECT STARCH COMBINING

The salivary enzyme that converts starch into sugar, known as ptyalin, is destroyed by acid. As we have said, if you eat starch with protein so that an acid juice is secreted, starch digestion is brought to a stop. Therefore, don't eat starches with acid fruits or with proteins.

Try this experiment. Take a dry starch such as oatmeal into your mouth. Notice that as you chew it and hold it in your mouth, it increases in bulk because it absorbs saliva. If you hold it long enough, it will become somewhat sweet, due to the conversion of starch into sugar by the ptyalin in your saliva. Now boil the oatmeal and put it into your mouth. Notice it will not increase in bulk because it cannot take up the saliva. Also, even though it is held for a prolonged period, it will not become sweet. This little experiment should reveal the importance of eating starch dry. When you eat soaked cereals or soups thickened with starch, the starch is not digested, so these make poor foods.

Oatmeal, cracked wheat or other cereals that have been soaked or boiled do not undergo salivary digestion even if they are eaten without milk and sugar. When you eat them with milk and sugar, digestion is doubly impossible. Sugar or honey partially or completely inhibit the secretion of ptyalin needed to digest the starch. The addition of sugar also induces overeating of starches.

When boiled cereals and sugars are hurried into the stomach without saliva, fermentation follows. Day-after-day gastrointestinal fermentation results from starch- and sugar-eating. Throat and nasal irritation, chronic irritation of the stomach, obesity, tonsillitis, arthritis, adenoids and other diseases may develop as a consequence of this constant fermentation. Dental decay also follows.

Oats seem to have the worst effect on the teeth. Wheat is the most acid-forming of the cereals. Rice, which is probably the best of the cereals, is the staple article of food in the diet of more than half of the people in the world. But cases of beri-beri in human beings have been reported even where whole and not polished rice constituted the bulk of the diet.

Never before in history has as much cereal grain and refined flour been consumed as in America and parts of Europe since the perfection of the rolling mill process in 1879. Cereal products and bread are consumed in enormous quantities, and a great deal of sickness results from these acid-forming foods.

The advocates of whole grains and whole wheat did their work too well. Vegetarians are usually great eaters of cereals. These people (who are more properly called *cerealists*) consume far too much cereal and suffer much because they eat their cereal in forms that ferment before they can be digested. These so-called "vegetarians" who eat large amounts of cereals would actually be harmed less by eating moderate amounts of meat.

Cereals are best omitted from the diet entirely and should be omitted especially from the diet of infants. The intestinal substances required for the digestion of starch are not secreted until a baby is about a year old. No starch, and especially no cereals, should be given to a child before he or she is two years old. For adults and children alike, sweet fruits are as nourishing as cereals and are easier to digest.

Any psychological or nutritional influence that devitalizes cell life and prevents ideal cell development reduces tissue development below the ideal and lays the foundation for degenerative diseases galore, not to mention excess weight. The indigestion and catarrh that result from eating cooked and soaked starches or eating sugar and starch together serve as starting points for the evolution of a whole series of later diseases. To remove the accumulated effects of obesity through dieting without removing the causes of poor digestion and assimilation is useless. Obesity and other diseases begin where cause begins and persist where cause persists.

RULES FOR CORRECT STARCH COMBINING

1. Eat starch and protein foods at separate meals.
2. Do not eat starches with fruits in any classifications (except the avocado), or with commercial sugars or honey.
3. Eat cereals dry—don't cook or soak them—to insure the conversion of starches into sugar.
4. Eat minimal amounts of cereals, for they do not form part of a natural diet.

MENUS FOR WEEK THREE
Spring and Summer
ADDING STARCH TO THE DIET

	Noon	*Evening*
MONDAY	cantaloupe (as much as desired)	vegetable salad* 1 or 2 baked potatoes unsalted butter

*Tomatoes or lemon juice (acids) should not be included in a salad that is followed by a starch.

	Noon	*Evening*
TUESDAY	½ pint strawberries 2 ounces walnuts and hazelnuts	vegetable salad steamed cauliflower
WEDNESDAY	1 or 2 mangos	vegetable salad 4 ounces steamed beets
THURSDAY	½ pint blueberries	vegetable salad ½ avocado 3 ounces brown rice
FRIDAY	*ripe* pineapple (as much as desired)	vegetable salad 2 ounces almonds
SATURDAY	½ pint blueberries 2 ounces pignolias	vegetable salad steamed corn
SUNDAY	watermelon (as much as desired)	vegetable salad 2 ounces cashews

MENUS FOR WEEK THREE

Fall and Winter

	Noon	*Evening*
MONDAY	honeydew melon (as much as desired)	vegetable salad 1 baked sweet potato

	Noon	*Evening*
TUESDAY	carrot juice 2 slices whole wheat bread* 1 small pat of unsalted butter	vegetable salad steamed broccoli
WEDNESDAY	1 papaya ½ avocado	vegetable salad 2 ounces almonds
THURSDAY	fruit salad 2 ounces black walnuts	vegetable salad 1 Jerusalem artichoke
FRIDAY	leafy green salad 1 grapefruit	vegetable salad 2 medium white potatoes 1 small pat of unsalted butter (optional)
SATURDAY	1 orange 2 ounces filberts or unprocessed raw milk cheese	vegetable salad yellow squash
SUNDAY	green beans 2 steamed Irish potatoes 1 small pat of unsalted butter	vegetable salad steamed kale

*The Hygienist omits bread entirely from the diet.

PART THREE

EATING FOR
THE HEALTH OF IT

However correct the quality of our food may be, if we habitually overeat, our whole nature is injured, and always in proportion to our excess.

SYLVESTER GRAHAM (1794–1851)
Pioneer Hygienist

CHAPTER NINE

THE MAINTENANCE PLAN: SLIMHOOD FOREVER

GOOD DIETS end sooner or later, and to be lastingly effective must be followed by a continued healthful eating pattern. If you did not reach your goal after following the three- (or four-) week program, follow the maintenance plan given in this chapter for one week and then begin the diet again. Repeat until you have reached your goal.

Although the following recipes are intended to be used on maintenance, some of them can be adjusted and used when you are losing weight. Just reduce the amount according to your needs. Be careful! Natural foods, just like processed and denatured foods, are fattening when eaten beyond your needs. Dieters never have a license to eat more than two ounces of nuts per day, more than one-half an avocado per day, or too many sweet fruits.

Whole raw foods should always be your first choice. These are nutritionally superior. To help satisfy your palate, however, the recipes provide a nice variation, although some of them may *sound* bland and dull to you until you try them. There's a reason for this. Hygienist Russell T. Trall, M.D. explains why ("The Hygienic Diet," *Dr. Shelton's Hygienic Review*, August 1974):

> If we view the "wholesome" foods recommended in the multitudinous cookbooks that flood the land, many of them prepared for and issued by the food manufacturers, you will look in vain for anything more than dietetic abominations. Thousands are ever busy inventing new recipes in cookery designed to pander to depraved appetites and to constantly mislead the world into bad and worse complications of highly seasoned and indigestible viands. Look through a hundred of the books that come from the press on the subject and you will scarcely find one recipe for a wholesome dish, or one line of sound advice. So far as the generalities of instruction contained in these books is concerned, the world would be as well off if these books had never been written.

In the nutritionally sound diet for the '80s and '90s found in this book, substitute the word "wholesome" for "bland" and "nutritious" for "dull." Change your mind-set and forget about highly seasoned, indigestible conglomerations. Keep meals simple. Try to vary your maintenance program by eating one cooked meal every other day, then one every three days. Remember that cooking impairs or destroys the protective and nutritive values of foods. Buying fruits and vegetables to provide minerals and vitamins for yourself or your family and then destroying the vitamins and extracting the minerals and throwing them away in the process of preparing the foods fails of its purpose. Only when you eat fruit uncooked and consume big salads of uncooked vegetables can you be sure of obtaining a sufficient supply of minerals and vitamins.

The nearer to their natural and unchanged state foods are eaten, the better they are for you. The natural affinity existing between the needs of your cells and the nutritional elements in natural foods gives you an infallible guarantee that you will get the needed salts, vitamins and other food elements from natural foods. All true foods are more tasty raw than cooked. Cooked food, sans seasoning, is flat and insipid, as well as less nutritious.

The following are some of the pluses of an uncooked diet:

1. Uncooked foods requiring more chewing, supply the teeth and gums with much-needed resistance exercise, thus forcing blood into the gum areas, which promotes oral health.

2. This necessary chewing also insures proper insalivation.

3. The necessity for chewing uncooked foods insures tasting them to the fullest, which in turn assures proper adaptation of internal digestive juices to the character of the food.

4. Chewing and tasting the food also tends to prevent overeating.

5. Uncooked foods preserve the mouth and stomach from the injury produced by hot foods.

6. Uncooked foods possess the proper proportion of nutritious and nonnutritious matter to which the anatomical construction and physiological powers of the alimentary organs of the human body are constitutionally adapted.

7. Eating uncooked foods tends to prevent pernicious food combinations.

8. Uncooked foods possess vitamins and minerals, enzymes, salts, acids, carbohydrates, proteins and fats in the organic and unimpaired state in which Nature produced them.

9. Uncooked foods are not so easily adulterated as are the canned, pickled, embalmed foods so widely eaten today.

10. Uncooked foods, if spoiled, cannot be camouflaged and passed off as good food the way cooked foods can be.

12. The uncooked diet saves time, food and labor in preparation.

You must understand that the following recipes for cooked food are to be used sparingly. Recipes where vegetables are steamed, baked, blended, cut and/or diced are always inferior to those using raw, whole foods. We recommend that you eat as many raw foods for meals or parts of meals as possible, but don't use them for snacks or desserts.

The compulsive overeater can overeat on raw foods and still lose weight, as long as no conventional food is taken. Because of their high nutritive and high fiber and water content (fruits and vegetables are 75 percent to 98 percent water), they will not cause weight gain.

FRUIT RECIPES

Mango Special (serves 1)

Cut a medium-sized mango in half, slicing over the large, flat seed. With a sharp paring knife, cut the meat of the mango into cubes. Arrange the cubes on a romaine lettuce leaf along with some raisins.

Recipe by Hygienist Joy Gross

Shalimar Breakfast (serves 1)

1–2 BANANAS   1 MANGO

Slice into large pieces. Top with 2–3 ounces of ground dates.*

Recipe by Hygienist Dr. Keki Sidhwa, D.O., N.D.

Fruit Salad (serves 1)

Use butter crunch lettuce as a base in an attractive medium salad bowl. Core a golden delicious apple and cut it into wedges, six or eight, depending on the size of the apple. Fan it out in a circle over the lettuce. Peel either one large or two medium kiwi fruits, slice them and place them over the apple wedges. Top with several Bing cherries.

This fruit salad can be preceded with a glass of red apple and celery juice.

Recipe by Hygienist Erma Benesh

Fruit Bouquet

APPLES (VARIETY)	GREEN GRAPES
PEARS (VARIETY)	AVOCADOS
RIBIER GRAPES	

*Be aware that the nutritional value of fruits decreases when they are ground, blended or sliced.

Wash all fruit, leave whole and dry. Arrange as desired in a large bowl or platter. Create your own fruit bouquet.

Recipe by Hygienist Helen Lamar

Fruit Sundae (serves 2)

½ CUP BLUEBERRIES   ½ CUP PINEAPPLE CUBES
½ CUP STRAWBERRIES   6 OUNCES SOFT RICOTTA CHEESE

Add the mixed fruit to a scoop of ricotta cheese. Place an extra large strawberry at the top of your sundae.

Recipe by Hygienist Sharon Dedinas, D.C.

PROTEIN COMBO RECIPES

Sunshine Salad (serves 1)

Use red leaf lettuce as a base for this colorful salad. Peel and seed a red or pink grapefruit and a large sweet navel orange. Slice them and layer one over the other in a pretty bowl. Add six large strawberries, surrounded with a ring of alfalfa sprouts. A rib of celery can be added to this salad. Serve 1 or 2 ounces of blanched almonds (see below) to complete the meal.

If a person does not find these salads satisfying at first, the amount of lettuce and sprouts can be increased.

Recipe by Hygienist Erma Benesh

Blanching Almonds Without Heat

Wash about two dozen almonds well and drain. Put in a glass jar. Sprinkle with water and remove excess liquid. Leave overnight, with jar tightly capped. In the morning the skins can be easily removed with your fingers. Thus, you avoid the harm of using heat.

Recipe by Hygienist Jo Willard

Stuffed Pepper Salad (serves 1)

Use the heart of endive for a green base on a lovely china salad plate. Wash a medium-size red pepper. Cut the top off, wash out the seeds and cut out the veins. Fill the cavity with grated zucchini and alfalfa sprouts or other sprouts of your choice. Top the pepper with two tablespoons of ground sunflower seeds. Serve with a rib of celery, including the tender leaves.

Recipe by Hygienist Erma Benesh

Almond Vegetable Dip* (serves 2)

Make ¼ cup of celery juice in a juicer and transfer it to a blender. Grind ½ cup of almonds in a nut grinder and add to blender. Liquefy blender contents on high speed, adding more juice or ground almonds until the desired consistency is reached.

Use as a vegetable dip.

Recipe by Hygienist Marty Wheeler

Orange Sherbet (serves 1)

2 ORANGES   6–8 ALMONDS

Blend one part blanched almonds with two parts pitted and peeled orange.

Recipe by Hygienist Gladys Aaron

Pineapple Ambrosia (serves 4)

1 RIPE PINEAPPLE   1 CUP SUNFLOWER SEEDS
½ CUP SESAME SEEDS   (quantities of seeds may vary to suit your taste)

*Whenever a recipe calls for grinding nuts, it must be remembered that this is certainly not the ideal way to eat nuts. *Chew* the nuts 90 percent of the time. Save ground nuts for special occasions.

Prepare and blend pineapple in blender or food processor. Remove from blender and pour into large bowl. Add sunflower and sesame seeds and mix well. Place in small glass jars. Soak overnight. The dormant seeds start to activate due to the bromelain enzyme in the pineapple, making the food more easily digestible. Use for breakfast, lunch or supper.

Chew slowly, thoroughly and lovingly. Food creates new cells for your eyes, your toes or your nose. Have reverence for it.

Recipe by Hygienist Jo Willard

Coconut Breakfast (serves 1)

1 LARGE SLICE OF PINEAPPLE   2–4 OUNCES GRATED FRESH COCONUT
2 SLICED ORANGES

Sprinkle coconut over fruit.

Recipe by Hygienist William Esser, D.C., N.D.

VEGETABLE RECIPES

Vegetable Bouquet

1 BUNCH EACH OF CARROTS,   2 CUCUMBERS
    CELERY AND BROCCOLI   2 RED PEPPERS
1 CAULIFLOWER   2 GREEN PEPPERS

Wash all vegetables, leave whole and dry. Arrange as desired in a decorative platter or dish and garnish with parsley. Create your own bouquet.

Recipe by Hygienist Helen Lamar

Eggplant Casserole Supreme (serves 2)

6 TOMATOES   ½ GREEN PEPPER
1 EGGPLANT   PARSLEY

Cut up six peeled tomatoes, parsley, ½ green pepper, and one eggplant (diced). Steam until eggplant is

::::::::::::::::::::::::::::::

tender. Place in baking casserole and bake about 10 minutes at 400 degrees. Remove from oven and top with 4 ounces of ground nuts.

Recipe by Hygienist Dorthy K. Brosious

Blended Salad (1 serving, 8 to 12 ounces)

½ TOMATO
½ CUCUMBER
½ RED OR GREEN PEPPER

3 TO 4 LEAVES ROMAINE LETTUCE
2 CELERY STALKS

Use blender or food processor to blend.

Recipe by Hygienist Christopher Gian-Cursio, N.D., D.C.

Hygienic Tacos and Guacamole

LETTUCE LEAVES (romaine or leaf are best)
FILLINGS (Hygienic Guacamole)

AVOCADO SLICES
ALFALFA SPROUTS
TOMATOES

Wash lettuce leaves, dry in a spin dryer or between towels, and serve on a large plate or platter. Prepare fillings (see below) and offer them on plates and in bowls. Put out an empty plate for each guest to assemble his own taco as he observes you assemble yours. Assemble tacos by first putting a lettuce leaf on a plate (use two leaves if one has any tears or holes). Then place the Hygienic Guacamole lengthwise down the middle of the lettuce leaf, and add avocado slices, tomato slices and sprouts.

To eat tacos, use your hands. (Tacos are sandwiches!) Simply fold over the two long sides, holding the sandwich together so that it resembles a Mexican taco.

Hygienic Guacamole (serves 2)

3 AVOCADOS   2 TOMATOES
¼ LEMON OR LIME   2 STALKS CELERY
¼ GRAPEFRUIT

Halve avocados and scoop flesh into a bowl. Using a fork, mash avocado, leaving it somewhat chunky. Juice lemon or lime and grapefruit and add juices to bowl.

Wash and dice tomatoes (halve or quarter cherry tomatoes). Wash celery, cut off and discard leaves and dice finely. Mix together with the avocados.

These Hygienic Tacos have been a big hit among everyone we served them to. They are more fun, more delicious, and easier than cut-up salads. People enjoy making their own tacos from the fixings you put on the table.

Recipe by Hygienist Marty Wheeler

Mixed Green Salad (serves 1)

Use crisp, dark green romaine lettuce as a base for this hearty salad. Slice a medium cucumber (use the peeling if it is not waxed), large ripe tomato, and ½ of a ripe avocado. Arrange pleasingly. Grate a medium carrot for color and top with bean sprouts.

This salad can be preceded by a glass of carrot and celery juice.

Recipe by Hygienist Erma Benesh

STARCH AND MILDLY STARCHY RECIPES

Wild Rice (serves 1)

2 CUPS CELERY JUICE   1 CUP WILD RICE (for economy,
                                mix with brown rice)

Bring celery juice and rice up to a boil with lid off for four minutes. Put lid on, turn down heat and cook for forty to fifty minutes. For the last ten minutes, turn off heat. If desired, add a nonstarch steamed vegetable such as string beans or zucchini. Add unsalted butter or mashed avocado.

Recipe by Hygienist Ruth Huberman

Cauliflower Supreme (serves 4)

1 HEAD CAULIFLOWER   ¼ CUP UNSALTED BUTTER

Steam cauliflower whole and spoon the unsalted butter over the top just before serving. Serve after a large green salad course with a steamed green vegetable.

Recipe by Hygienist Effie Troyer

Stuffed Peppers with Corn (serves 3)

6 PEPPERS   1 CUP DICED CELERY
3 CUPS FRESH CORN KERNELS   3 TABLESPOONS CHOPPED PARSLEY

Slice top from stem side of peppers. Steam peppers about five minutes. In the meantime, cut corn kernels from fresh cobs. Mix corn with celery and parsley and fill the steamed peppers. Drop a dab of unsalted butter on the top of each pepper and bake for about thirty minutes. (Peppers stuffed with brown rice can be made in a similar way).

Recipe by Hygienist Jack Trop

Baked Corn

Preheat oven to 400 degrees.

Remove silk tassel from corn ears. Replace corn husks round corn. Place ears under running water and shake off excess water. Put ears on rack in oven and bake for 10 to 15 minutes. Excellent for picnics—you peel your own corn.

An alternate method is to cook the corn in its

husks in boiling water for 6 minutes. The corn silk peels right off with the husk and the corn is juicier than if cooked by the old prehusked method.

Recipe by Hygienist Dorthy K. Brosious

Carrot and Celery Shangri-La (serves 3)

2 CUPS CARROTS,
  sliced ⅛ to ¼ inch thick
2 CUPS CELERY,
  sliced diagonally, ⅛ to
  ¼-inch thick

DRIED PARSLEY, if desired
UNSALTED BUTTER, if desired

Steam vegetables until tender. Add butter just before serving. Serve after a large salad with a potato, if desired.

Recipe by Hygienist Frances Cheatham

MENUS FOR MAINTENANCE

Spring and Summer

SLIMHOOD FOREVER

Morning	*Noon*	*Evening*
MONDAY		
pineapple (as much as desired) 2 ounces sunflower seeds (if well tolerated)	vegetable salad collards yellow squash	vegetable salad beet greens unprocessed raw milk cheese (2 ounces) or ½ avocado
TUESDAY		
watermelon (as much as desired) (not for hypo-glycemics)*	4 ounces grapes 1 papaya celery ½ or 1 small avocado	vegetable salad green squash spinach almonds (2 ounces)

*Hypoglycemics must adjust the Maintenance Plan to their specific needs.

Morning	*Noon*	*Evening*

WEDNESDAY
fresh figs
peaches
apricots (as many
  as desired)

leafy salad
green peas
carrots
parsnips

vegetable salad
cabbage
spinach
unprocessed raw
  milk cheese
  (2 ounces) or
  ½ avocado

THURSDAY
strawberries
1 grapefruit
2 ounces almonds

leafy salad
baked corn on cob
(recipe page 127)

vegetable salad
broccoli
green beans
sunflower seeds
  (2 ounces)
  (if seeds are
  well tolerated)

FRIDAY
1 muskmelon

Joy's Mango
Special (recipe
page 121)

vegetable salad
asparagus
broccoli

SATURDAY
½ pint blueberries
1 orange
2 ounces pecans

Bing cherries
raspberries (as
  many as desired)
celery
½ avocado

vegetable salad
unprocessed raw
  milk cheese (2
  ounces) or
avocado or seeds

SUNDAY
2 peaches
6 dates

Helen's Fruit
Bouquet (recipe
page 121)

vegetable salad
chard
cashews (2 ounces)

MENUS FOR MAINTENANCE

Fall and Winter

SLIMHOOD FOREVER

Morning	*Noon*	*Evening*
MONDAY		
1 grapefruit	1 apple	vegetable salad
2 oranges	1 pear	broccoli
	½ or 1 small	string beans
	avocado	pecans and walnuts
		(2 ounces)
TUESDAY		
raisins	spinach salad	vegetable salad
(unsulfured)	carrots	brussels sprouts
dried figs	napa cabbage	cabbage
apricots (as many		macadamia nuts
as desired)		(2 ounces) or ½
		avocado or seeds
WEDNESDAY		
honeydew melon	leafy salad	Helen's Vegetable
(as much as	cauliflower	Bouquet (recipe
desired)	Chinese cabbage	page 124)
	yams	
THURSDAY		
dates	vegetable salad	fruit salad
2 bananas (not	collards	
for hypo-	filberts	
glycemics)	(2 ounces) or ½	
	avocado or seeds	

Morning	*Noon*	*Evening*
FRIDAY		
1 orange	spinach salad	vegetable salad
1 grapefruit	apple	mustard greens
walnuts	½ or 1 avocado	red cabbage
(2 ounces)		pistachio nuts
		(2 ounces)
SATURDAY		
4 figs	1–2 oranges	Marty's Hygienic
1 banana	1 slice pineapple	Tacos (recipe
	unprocessed raw	page 125)
	milk cheese (2	
	ounces) or ½	
	avocado or seeds	
SUNDAY		
2 apples	vegetable salad	vegetable salad
1 persimmon	yellow wax beans	bamboo sprouts
	kale	green squash
	steamed sweet	brazil nuts
	potatoes with	(4 ounces)
	unsalted butter	

I saw few die of hunger—of eating, a hundred thousand.

BENJAMIN FRANKLIN (1706–1790)

::

CHAPTER TEN

LIVING THE SLIM LIFE

YOU HAVE EMBARKED on an exciting and exhilarating journey toward reaching your potential. It will lead you to greater understanding of your body and mind, setting you on an ascending path of health and leading to development of your highest potential.

There is a societal preoccupation today with the superficial appearance of the body. "Thin" bodies are "in." Not all of us can achieve "thinness" as prescribed by Madison Avenue. This can be frustrating, but has little relevance to happiness and health.

Each person has a different bone structure and anatomy, as well as a different chemistry that may not be able to meet these so-called standards of slimness. Don't cultivate an impossible ideal based on the slick advertising yardsticks, or you will view your body as totally inadequate and beyond change or repair. Why strive to match that madness and lose hope? The reality is that an advertising image had nothing to do with your evolvement, with your search for health and happiness, with your need to be loved or your need for emotional, intellectual and spiritual growth.

You are a perfect human being as you are. Unless you realize that you are the total reality of your cultural patterns, your education, your memory and the social mores you have been taught, no change can take place.

AWARENESS OF WHAT IS FIT FOOD FOR HUMANITY IS KEY

Be aware that distress, negative emotions and lack of inner peace are not conducive to change.

Be aware that your body does indeed change with time and that you must not be continually preoccupied with it because it is your *mind* that sets the guidelines and allows your body to change within those guidelines.

Your body seeks overall comfort. Gentle, loving, consistent discipline will keep it comfortable. The Hygienic Diet is ideal for enabling both mind and body to reach perfect harmony when it is used in conjunction with all of the prerequisites for health that affect both the body and the mind, including sunshine, fresh, clean air, adequate rest and sleep, clean, unadulterated water, emotional poise and activity.

To avoid being trapped in societal garbage, never view your body as an entity in itself; see it as one aspect of an entire human being.

Peace is found in harmony, in understanding your personal parameters and limitations, in expanding consciousness and in knowing that discipline is not deprivation but living in harmony with the Laws of Nature.

You are what you believe, what you perceive, what

you think. You constantly reinforce these beliefs with your speech. "I am a compulsive overeater" reinforces this in your subconscious. If that thought arises, change it to "I *was* a compulsive overeater" and add, "I am a beautiful being to be loved and cared for." Change "I love spaghetti and meatballs" to "Spaghetti with tomato sauce contains irritating spices, overprocessed starches and highly acidic cooked tomatoes which will engorge my beautiful body and cause illness." "One of my favorite foods is chocolate" (or whatever) reinforces *that* habit into your subconscious. You now have new knowledge, new perceptions, new goals: HEALTH. Think "Chocolate contains theobromides, caffeine and high sugar. It is a poison. I will not violate my beautiful body."

Once you begin to realize the effects of perception—or how you view people, food, animals and life itself—you can mold new thoughts and begin to grow and evolve emotionally, intellectually and spiritually. You no longer are stuck in the mire of the destructive thoughts, habits and speech patterns you accepted previously.

Growth and change will accelerate and a beautiful flowering of your potentials will manifest itself. Only joy and happiness can result from these changes.

New consciousness awakens you, new attitudes inspire you. What power, to become aware of how a thought can affect the chemistry of your body! Resolve to become sensitized to the power of thought.

Your mind touches every cell of your body. As you take charge of your thoughts and change poor habits into good habits, you will realize that all obstacles of

:::::::::::::::::::::::::::::

sickness are removed. Superior health and happiness are under *your* control. You are in charge.
Take this responsibility into your own hands!

SECRETS OF SUCCESS

Whether you change your eating patterns, your general lifestyle or your job, or when changes perceived as losses occur, you must see each change as part of the evolutionary process—like summer moving into autumn, like winter gliding into spring. These are all part of the natural flow of life. They should be viewed as opportunities to grow, mature and evolve.

Find a commitment which transcends you. The outcome of health and life itself depends greatly on the nature and quality of your thoughts.

With improved health comes the glorious feeling of having control over your life and greater influence in confronting all of life's contingencies.

Not only will you experience the joy of living, adding years to your life, but you will realize that the *quality of life* is the key to your time on this planet. Quality time is joyous time!

Love yourself. You are very beautiful.

APPENDICES

Appendix A

CORRECT FOOD COMBINING

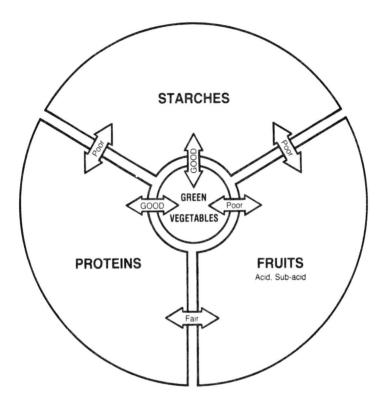

Exceptions: Tomatoes should not be eaten with starches (because tomatoes contain acids). Ideally, melons and milk should each be taken alone. Sweet fruits, which are not included in the diagram, may be combined with sub-acid fruits and neutral vegetables. The avocado combines well with all foods except proteins and melons.

Hygienic books may be obtained from the following:

NATURAL HYGIENE, INC.
P.O. Box 2132
Huntington Station
Shelton, CT 06484

SHELTON'S BOOKS
121 Marcia Place
San Antonio, TX 78209

WILLOW PUBLISHING, INC.
Box 6636 AH
San Antonio, TX 78209-6636

THE AMERICAN NATURAL HYGIENE SOCIETY, INC.
12816 Race Track Road
Tampa, FL 33625

COLLEGE OF LIFE SCIENCE
6600 D Burleson Road
Austin, TX 78744

HEALTH RESEARCH
P.O. Box 70
Mokelumne Hill, CA 95245

GLOSSARY

Acid: A chemical containing hydrogen replaceable by a metal to form a salt. Acids are sour in taste, corrosive, and soluble in water.

Albumin: An important protein component found in animal and vegetable tissue.

Alkaline: The opposite of acid, containing more hydroxyl than hydrogen ions.

Amino acids: Organic compounds necessary for the maintenance of life. They represent an end product of protein metabolism.

Antidote: Anything that counteracts an injurious effect.

Arteriosclerosis: Hardening of the arteries.

Assimilation: The change of digested food into parts of the living organism.

Blood: The fluid traveling throughout the body that brings nutriment and oxygen to all tissues and transports away carbon dioxide and other waste products.

Caffeine: A bitter white alkaloid derived from coffee, tea and kola nuts, and used as a diuretic or stimulant.

Calcium: A brilliant, silver-white metal characterized by a strong affinity for oxygen. It is an abundant and widely distributed element.

Carbohydrate: A food in the sugar or starch family.

Catarrh: Inflammation of mucous membranes, especially of the nose and throat.

Cholesterol: A waxy alcohol found in egg yolks, meat, fish (particularly organ meats and shellfish), animal fats, and dairy products such as butter, cheese, cream and milk.

Circulation: The passage of blood from the heart to all parts of the body and its return from the tissues to the heart.

Cirrhosis: An inflammatory disease of the liver involving the replacement of liver cells by fibrous tissue.

Compulsive overeater: A person whose pattern of overeating is uncontrolled; the habit is repeated over and over again.

Denatured foods: Inferior foods that have been impaired or altered by processing and are not in the state Nature prepared them.

Digestion: The process of breaking down food so that it can be absorbed through the lining of the intestinal tract.

Distilled water: Water that has been obtained by the process of vaporizing and then condensing the vapor.

Diuretics: Drugs or substances that stimulate kidney function.

Enzymes: Any of numerous proteins or conjugated proteins produced by living organisms and functioning as biochemical catalysts in living organisms.

Fasting: Rest: physically, psychologically and physiologically (abstinence from food except for drinking *pure* water).

Fats: Compounds of glycerol and fatty acids. Each fat molecule contains polyunsaturated, monounsaturated or saturated fatty acids in varying proportions, depending upon the type of fat.

Formic acid: A preservative found in honey that hinders its digestion.

Hygienist: One who lives by Nature's laws: natural foods from the earth and trees, fresh air, fresh water, rest, sunshine, emotional poise, activity and awareness of biochemical individuality.

Hypoglycemia: The presence of too little sugar in the blood.

Inflammation: The reaction of tissues to injury.

Irritant: Anything that interferes with the normal activity of some vital process or organ.

Metabolism: The body's utilization of the sugars, proteins and fats to maintain proper weight and body functioning.

Minerals: Chemical compounds not containing carbon found in Nature; some are necessary for the maintenance of life.

Mono-meal: A meal consisting of a single food.

Necrotizing enterocolitis: Inflammation of the small and large intestine with tissue damage.

Neonatal hypothyroidism: Underactivity of the thyroid gland in the newborn.

Nutrition: The sum total of all the processes of digestion and utilization by which food is changed to living tissues.

Oxygen: An essential ingredient for life, which is present in the blood and nourishes all parts of the body.

Pepsin: A digestive enzyme found in gastric juice.

Poison: A drug or other substance very dangerous to health and life.

Polyunsaturated fats: Fats that are liquid at room temperature. They include such oils as corn, safflower, soybean, sunflower, walnut and sesame.

Proteins: A basic food substance containing nitrogen; characteristic constituents of all living matter.

Protoplasm: The necessary materials that constitute living cells.

Ptyalin: The salivary enzyme that converts starch into sugar.

Pyridine: A flammable, colorless or yellowish liquid base used as a solvent, as a denaturant for alcohol, and to synthesize vitamins and drugs.

Saturated fats: Fats that are solid at room temperature. They can be found in both plant and animal foods, including meat fat (lard, salt pork, suet, bacon fat), butter, coconut, and vegetable shortening.

Toxins: Poisonous products in the blood which result in illness.

Uric acid: A substance found in the blood and urine that is formed in the body as a waste product of protein metabolism.

Vegetarian: A person who eats fruits, vegetables and legumes but no meat.

Vitamins: Any of the various organic substances that are essential for the maintenance of normal health.

Bibliography

Atkins, Robert C. *Dr. Atkins' Nutrition Breakthrough.* New York: Bantam Books, 1981.

Baker, Samm Sinclair and Sylvia Schur. *The Delicious Quick-Trim Diet.* New York: Villard Books, 1983.

Bidwell, Vickey. "Success, At Last!" *Natural Weight-Loss Newsletter* (1984).

Brownell, Kelly D. *The Partnership Diet Program.* New York: Rawson, Wade Publishers, Inc., 1980.

Burton, Alec. "Milk," *Dr. Shelton's Hygienic Review* (vol. XXXV, no. 11, 1974).

Coco, James, and Marion Paone. *The James Coco Diet.* New York: Bantam Books, 1984.

Cornaro, Luigi. *Discourses and Letters on a Sober and Temperate Life.* New York: Fowler and Wells, 1848.

Dewey, E. H. *The No-Breakfast Plan and the Fasting Cure.* London: L. N. Fowler & Co., 1900.

Doyle, Roger. *The Vegetarian Handbook.* New York: Crown Publishers, Inc., 1979.

Dyer, Wayne W. *Your Erroneous Zones.* New York: Avon Books, 1976.

Esser, William L. *Dictionary of Natural Foods.* Tampa Florida: Natural Hygiene Press, 1983.

Flatto, Edwin. "The Question, Box," *Herald of Health* (July 1974).

Flick, Frank. *Weight Control and Fitness: A Scientific Approach.* Bensenville, Illinois: Health & Education Services Corp., 1973.

Fox, Arnold. *The Beverly Hills Medical Diet.* New York: Bantam Books, 1981.

——. "Taking the Bite Out of Cancer," *Let's Live* (September 1983).

Fry, T.C. and Vickey Bidwell. "Why We Become Overweight," *Life Science* (1984).

Gaev, Dorothy M. "Ten Ways to Slow the Aging Process," *Total Health* (November 1983).

Goldbeck, Nikki and David. *The Dieter's Companion.* New York: McGraw-Hill Book Co., 1975.

Goodman, David. "Breaking the Protein Myth," *Whole Life Times* (July/August 1984).

Goulart, Frances Sheridan. "Vitamins and Mineral Companions," *Total Health* (May 1984).

Graham, Sylvester. *Lectures on the Science of Human Life.* Boston: Marsh, Copen, Lyon & Webb, 1839.

Grommet, Janet K. "How to Diet Less & Lose More," *Bottom Line* (30 January 1985).

Gross, Joy. *The 30-Day Way to a Born-Again-Body.* New York: Rawson, Wade, Inc., 1978.

——. *The Vegetarian Child.* Secaucus, New Jersey: Lyle Stuart, Inc., 1983.

——. *Thin Again: Improved Fitness in 30 Days.*

Guerra, Luis A. *The Bio-Diet.* New York: Crown Publishers, Inc., 1982.

Haas, Robert. *Eat to Win*. New York: Charles Scribner's Sons, 1984.

Henig, Robin. "Eat Right and Live Longer," CBS Publications, the Consumer Publishing Division of CBS Inc., 1983).

Holzman, David. "The Unknowns in Coffee," *Washington Post* (6 January 1985).

Katahn, Martin. *The 200 Calorie Solution*. New York: W. W. Norton & Co., Inc., 1982.

Kordel, Lelord. *Eat and Grow Slender*. New York: Macfadden-Bartell Corp., 1964.

Lloyd, Douglas S. "Questions for Passive Smokers," *Bridgeport (Conn.) Post* (7 February 1981).

Mason, Jim. "Natural Hygienist: Jo Willard," *Vegetarian Times* (February 1985).

—— and Peter Singer. *Animal Factories*. New York: Crown Publishers, Inc., 1980.

Mazel, Judy. *The Beverly Hills Diet*. New York: Berkley Publishing Group, 1981.

——. *The Beverly Hills Diet Lifetime Plan*. New York: Macmillan Publishing Co., Inc., 1982.

McDougall, John and Mary McDougall. "The Latest Thinking on Protein," *Vegetarian Times* (August 1984).

McGuire, Rick. "The Losing Battle: An Overview," *Total Health* (March 1984).

Mendelsohn, Robert S. "Nutrition," *The People's Doctor* (vol. 7, no. 1, 1981).

——. *Male Practice: How Doctors Manipulate Women*. Chicago: Contemporary Books, Inc., 1981.

Mirkin, Gabe with Laura Foreman. *Getting Thin*. Boston: Little, Brown and Co., Inc., 1983.

Morales, Betty Lee. "The Free Radical—The Common Denominator of Disease," *Let's Live* (July 1982).

Null, Gary and Staff. *Food Combining Handbook*. New York: Jove Publications, Inc., 1973.

Orbach, Susie. *Fat is a Feminist Issue*. New York: Berkley Publishing Group, 1978.

Pratt, Foster J. "The Three Kinds of Aging," *Modern Maturity* (December/January 1973–74).

Price, John F. and Clarence D. Brinson. *The Food of Geniuses*. Chicago: The Vegetarian Health Society, 1982.

Pritikin, Nathan. *The Pritikin Promise: 28 Days to a Longer, Healthier Life*. New York: Simon & Schuster, Inc. 1983.

Reuben, David. *Save Your Life Diet*. New York: Ballantine Books, 1975.

Rubin, Theodore Isaac. *The Thin Book by a Formerly Fat Psychiatrist*. New York: Simon & Schuster, Inc., 1967.

Sabatino, Frank D. "The White Plague," *Dr. Shelton's Hygienic Review* (July, 1979).

Schmeck, Harold M. Jr. "By Training the Brain Scientists Find Links to Immune Defenses," *New York Times* (1 Jan. 1985).

Sidhwa, Keki R. "Water-logged Tissues," *Dr. Shelton's Hygienic Review* (vol XXVI, no. 1, 1964).

Simone, Charles B. *Cancer and Nutrition*. New York: McGraw-Hill Book Co., 1983.

Shelton, Herbert M. *Food and Feeding*. Oklahoma City: How to Live Publishing Co., 1926.

——. *Human Life: Its Philosophy and Laws*. Oklahoma City: How to Live Publishing Co., 1928.

——. *The Hygienic System—Orthotrophy*. San Antonio: Dr. Shelton's Health School, 1935.

——. *Superior Nutrition*. San Antonio: Dr. Shelton's Health School, 1951.

:::::::::::::::::::::::::

———. *Human Beauty: Its Culture and Hygiene.* San Antonio: Dr. Shelton's Health School, 1958.

———. *Fasting Can Save Your Life.* Chicago: Natural Hygiene Press, 1964.

———. *Health for the Millions.* Chicago: Natural Hygiene Press, 1968.

———. *Food Combining Made Easy.* San Antonio: Willow Publishing Inc., 1982.

——— and Jean A. Oswald. *Fasting for the Health of It.* San Antonio: Willow Publishing, Inc., 1983.

Smith, Lendon. *Feed Yourself Right.* New York: McGraw-Mill Book Co., 1983.

Tilden, John H. *Food.* Denver: J. H. Tilden, 1916.

Trall, Russel T. *Hygienic Handbook.* New York: Samuel R. Wells Publishing, 1873.

Trop, Jack Dunn. *You Don't Have to Be Sick.* New York: Julian Press, 1961.

Wade, Carlson. *Health Foods Cookbook.* West Nyack, New York: Parker Publishing Co., Inc., 1969.

Warmbrand, Max. *Eat Well to Keep Well.* New York: Pyramid Publications, Inc., 1970.

Wells, Cliff. "Coffee: The Popular Poison," *Public Scrutiny.* (December 1979).

Williams, Roger J. *Nutrition Against Disease.* New York: Pitman Publications Corp., 1971.

Winter, Ruth, "Living Indefinitely," *New Woman* (July/August (1974).

Yiamouyiannis, John. *The Aging Factor.* Delaware, Ohio: Health Action Press., 1983.

INDEX

INDEX

Pineapple ambrosia, 123
Polyunsaturated fats, 43
Potato starch, 107
Premature aging, undigested proteins and, 32
Protein(s), 23, 95–106
  excess of, 32, 97
  rules for combining, 101–102
  sources of, 96
  undigested, 32, 96
Protein combo recipes, 122–124
Protein menus, Week Two
  fall and winter, 104–105
  spring and summer, 103–104
Ptyalin, 48–109
Pyridine, 56

Quality of life, 135

Radish tops, 85
Raw foods, 36
Rest, 18–19, 70
Roughage, 83

Salad(s), 83
  avocado, 72
  blended, 125
  green leafy, 84
  mixed green, 126
Salad dressings, 88
Salad recipes, 87–88
Salt, 41–43
Salt intoxication, 43
Saturated fried fats, 43–45
Self-destructive habits, 5, 7–8
Self-image, 7
Shalimar breakfast, 121
Sleep, 18–19. See also Rest
Spinach, 86
Spiritual maladjustment, 6
Starch(es), 76, 107–115
  classification of, 108
  correct combining, 109–111
  digestion of, 48
  rules for correct combining, 111
Starch foods, 107
Starch menus, Week Three
  fall and winter, 112–113
  spring and summer, 111–112
Starch and mildly starchy recipes, 126–128
Steaming chart
  starches, 108
  vegetables, 89–90
Stomach cancer, cooking oils and, 44–45
Strident voice, 10
Stuffed pepper salad, 123

Sub-acid fruits, 77
Success, secrets of, 135
Sunbaths, 19–20, 69
Sunshine, 16
Sunshine salad, 122
Sweet fruits, 78

Tacos, 125
Tannic acid, 56
Tars, 45–46
Tea, 56–57
Tears, 42
Tobacco, 46–48
Tomato(es), 75
Tomato and celery juice, 72
Tomato dressing, 89
Total fast, 67–71
Toxins, elimination of, 67, 97
Tryptophan, 60
Tumors
  tar and, 46
  undigested proteins and, 32
Turnip tops, 85, 86

Uncooked diet, pluses, 119–120
Unhappiness, 9

Vegans, 31
Vegetable bouquet, 124
Vegetable juices, 57, 72
Vegetables, 83–94
  acidic and alkaline, 28
  chopping, 87
  green leafy, 85
  neutral, 90–91
  nutritional value, 85
  raw, for salads, 88
  recipes, 124–126
  rules for eating, 90
  soaking in water, 86
  steamed, 89
Vegetarianism, 32
Vegetarians, 110. See also Vegans
Vinegar, 48–49
Vitamin D, 19
Vitamins, in fruits and vegetables, 74–76, 85, 86

Waste, adequate disposal of, 16
Water, 16, 51–54
  distilled, 67–68
  effect on digestive juices, 54
  excessive drinking of, 52–53
  important functions of, 51–52
Weighing in, 23–24
"White plague," 42
Wild rice, 126
Wound healing, 12

From the Book Brown Bozwell
a Stay Well Pg. 41 Tomatoes may be Com
bined with Low-Starchy Vegetables Like
Potatoes, Lima beans yams Carrots, beets
bee
grain, Winter squash. also Nuts & avocado
Rice